The Reboot wit

Juice D
Recipe Book

The Reboot with Joe
Juice Diet
Recipe Book

Joe Cross

HODDER &
STOUGHTON

First published in Great Britain in 2014 by Hodder & Stoughton
An Hachette UK company

This edition published in 2017 by Hodder & Stoughton
An Hachette UK company

1

A CIP catalogue record for this title
is available from the British Library

Paperback ISBN 978 1 444 79835 7
Ebook ISBN 978 1 444 79834 0

Typeset in Scala and AG Book Rounded by
Palimpsest Book Production Limited, Falkirk, Stirlingshire

Printed and bound by CPI Group (UK) Ltd, Croydon, CRO 4YY

Hodder & Stoughton policy is to use papers that are
natural, renewable and recyclable products and made from
wood grown in sustainable forests. The logging and
manufacturing processes are expected to conform to the
environmental regulations of the country of origin.

Hodder & Stoughton Ltd
Carmelite House
50 Victoria Embankment
London EC4Y 0DZ
www.hodder.co.uk

Contents

Acknowledgements

Thank you to the Reboot Team – Kari Thorstensen, Amie Hannon, Brenna Ryan, Jamie Schneider, Sophie Carrel, Chris Zilo, Ameet Matura, Alex Tibbetts, Erin Flowers, Sarah Mawson, Sean Frechette, Vernon Caldwell, Jamin Mendelsohn, Kurt Engfehr, Shane Hodson, Stacy Kennedy and Claire Georgiou – who regardless of their jobs all take delight in creating and taste testing new and delicious Reboot-friendly recipes. Their work is in these pages.

The Reboot with Joe Medical Advisory Board (in addition to Stacy Kennedy) – Ronald Penny MD, DSc, Carrie Diulus MD and Adrian Rawlinson MD – who continue to endorse and advocate Rebooting as an effective means to achieve weight loss and health and always endeavour to keep me straight on my facts.

Sarah Hammond and the team at Hodder & Stoughton for their suggestion to do this book and their guidance and enthusiasm in bringing it to market.

Introduction

Seventy per cent of all disease is caused by lifestyle choices.[1]

Let me say that again.

Seventy per cent of all disease is caused by lifestyle choices.

What are those 'choices', you ask? Well, the big three are whether or not you smoke, how much you exercise, and what you eat and drink. It's pretty clear that if you make good choices (don't smoke, exercise consistently, eat healthy foods), you'll be on the right side of the fight against disease. But sometimes making those good choices is harder than you think. It's become normal – average, even – to be overweight in our society. And it's become pretty average to be managing a chronic illness by taking medication. In that case, I was just an average bloke.

A few years ago, on the cusp of 40, I took a long, hard look in the mirror and wasn't pleased with what was looking back at me – a lifetime of not-good choices (ok, fine: pretty terrible choices) has taken their predictable toll – I was chronically ill and almost 100 lbs overweight. But instead of registering nothing but shock and horror, I saw a silver lining – it was 70 per cent likely that I had caused this myself. And if that were the case, I had a pretty good chance of fixing it myself, too. In order to do that, I needed to enlist the help of Mother Nature, so I decided to consume nothing but the juice of fresh fruits and vegetables for 60 days. I chronicled this in the documentary *Fat, Sick & Nearly Dead*.

I had created a vicious cycle for myself and as I stood there looking in the mirror on the eve of my milestone birthday, I realised that if I didn't make a radical change, I would squander the incredible gifts I had been given and wind up in an early grave. When it finally dawned on me that perhaps I was the problem let me tell you that was a pretty sobering moment – it's hard to acknowledge that you are the agent of your own destruction, and pretty embarrassing too.

I had turned my back on Mother Nature and ignored the simple but powerful lesson that we are taught as young children. *Eat your vegetables and fruits.* This may sound simplistic, but at the time I had only the most glancing relationship with green vegetables – they were the things I moved to the side to get to the things I actually wanted – and 'fruit' was most often the maraschino cherry atop a sundae or a handful of berries that were decorating a plate of *real* dessert. What if I took my consumption of fruits and vegetables from almost zero to 100 per cent? That would be a pretty straightforward experiment, and would yield a definitive conclusion, right? But how to do it? The thought of eating pounds and pounds of plant food every day was daunting and, as anyone who has known me for 10 minutes will attest, I'm a guy in a hurry. It occurred to me that the most speedy and efficient method of flooding my system with nutrients would be to juice vegetables and fruits and consume nothing but that juice for a period of time. It was my hope it would reboot my system and return me to the state of good health I had known as a boy.

By the end of my journey I was medication free, had lost the 100lbs of weight and felt absolutely like new. I'd been given a fresh lease on life, and I decided to use the extra time and energy I had to try to help people just like me to see that there was an effective, simple way to reclaim their wellbeing and vitality. The intervening few years have so far surpassed my expectations that it's almost comical. *Fat, Sick & Nearly Dead* has, at the time of this writing, been seen by more than 11 million people around the world. My efforts to spread information and encouragement coalesced into a business and an online community, Reboot with Joe (www.rebootwithjoe.com), where millions of people have received the tools, recipes and community they needed to Reboot their lives. I've lectured all over the world and have been moved, inspired and humbled by the stories of personal transformation that people from Auckland to Oakland have shared with me.

My last book, *The Reboot with Joe Juice Diet*, became a great success very quickly, in part because people who had been inspired by the film wanted to know how they could fit the plan I followed to their own lives. We put together a group of plans that offered different ways to Reboot, allowing people to choose the Reboot plan that best suited their lifestyle. Now, one of the advantages of having an online community is that you get customer feedback immediately and without a filter. What I started to hear from Rebooters (I reckon you may be one of them!) who had followed the plans in my How-To book was twofold:

The first? 'More, please.'

So I've written this book for those of you that want *more* – more recipes, more support, more information and more variety. Whether it's your first Reboot, or your fourteenth, what you're about to read will help you re-set your palate, clear away the cobwebs and take responsibility for your health and wellbeing. And you'll find that this information has value beyond the period of your Reboot – I think it will help you incorporate the behaviours, recipes and choices that make this lifestyle permanent. This book is a companion to your Reboot plan (if you don't have one, pick up a copy of the *The Reboot with Joe Juice Diet* book or visit www. rebootwithjoe.com). You can use all of the recipes within this book as a substitute for the recipes on the Reboot plans – so you can customise your period of entirely plant-based eating and juicing to your taste! We've even colour-coded them to ensure that with any substitutions you are still getting a variety of vitamins and minerals. You can also take into account any health conditions, since we've listed those that are improved by a particular juice next to the relevant recipe. And if you're post Reboot, well, I reckon these are just great recipes to have on hand to combine with your favourite healthy grains or meat, or to enjoy on their own!

And the next is, 'What now?'

Well, my answer to 'What now' is *Fat, Sick & Nearly Dead 2,* released in the autumn of 2014. It addresses the next stage of the lifelong journey that follows a decision to change – one that I'm excited to share with you. If you want to find out how to see the film, be sure to visit us at www.rebootwithjoe.com and sign up for our newsletter.

You see, I got lucky. I stumbled onto a simple solution that had profound results. As far as I'm concerned, Rebooting saved my life – not just by adding years to my life but by returning me to a state of being that is characterised more by joy than despair, and by a sense of possibility far more potent than the threat of a doomed ending. And it can do the same for you, if you're lucky. I have a saying: 'Lady Luck follows a person of action'. I hope this book helps you take action.

Juice on!

How to use this book

This book is meant to accompany a Reboot – a period of time in which you consume only fresh fruits and vegetables. I am assuming that you have already decided on a Reboot plan and are already Rebooting or ready to go. If you don't have a plan, you can find some, for free, on my website www.rebootwithjoe.com. These same plans, along with tons of information about how Rebooting works and how to successfully Reboot, are also available in my book *The Reboot with Joe Juice Diet*.

I hope this new recipe book will provide inspiration to you and help keep your Reboot fresh and interesting. You may be tired of drinking my Mean Green juice, or maybe you really are not a fan of the Roasted Acorn Squash Stuffed with Mushrooms. That's OK. This recipe book will provide you with additional recipes that you can substitute for any of those on the Reboot plans, enabling you to customise your Reboot to your liking or to include what is seasonally fresh and available.

You can substitute any smoothie for one listed in the book, or any salad for another salad recipe here, and so on. For juices, we've colour-coded the juices – red, orange, green, purple and yellow. Try substituting with a like colour to make sure you are getting a variety of vitamins and minerals. If you have a health condition, pay attention to those listed by the recipe – this tells you which juices are particularly helpful for each condition. If you have diabetes or a thyroid condition, extra care should be taken when eating raw juice and foods; please check out the sections on Rebooting with Diabetes and Rebooting for Thyroid Conditions for more information.

And if you're not Rebooting? The recipes in this book are an excellent way to keep your diet full of fruits and veggies. So feel free to combine them with your favourite grains and meat, or enjoy the mains for a meatless feast.

The recipes here are a collection of old favourites as well as some new ones that we created just for this book. For more recipe inspiration, community and tools to help you with your Reboot, check out www.rebootwithjoe.com.

Key

Colour Try to drink a variety of colours. Substitute like colour for like colour on a Reboot plan.

Season The ideal season in the UK for one or more key items in this recipe to help you get produce at its best.

R Appropriate for a Reboot (which all recipes in this book are except for some of the pulp recipes).

⊘ This is a quick and easy item to make, using few ingredients and no elaborate preparation.

🏃 Great for post-workout – or if it's a juice, even during your workout.

✚ Especially helpful if you have one or more of the listed health conditions.

Reboot Daily Guide

On juicing-only days your fluid intake should look like this. Substitute other juices based on the colour indicated next to the recipe.

- **Wake up:** 9fl oz/250ml hot water with lemon and/or ginger
- **Breakfast:** Go Orange or Red
- **Mid-morning:** 16fl oz/500ml coconut water
- **Lunch:** Go Green
- **Afternoon snack:** Go Yellow or Red
- **Dinner:** Go Green
- **Dessert:** Go Purple or Orange
- **Bedtime:** Herbal tea
- **Throughout the day:** Drink lots of water (48fl oz/1.5 litres)

JUICING

How to make a juice

Wash produce thoroughly. Unwashed fruit and vegetables can be contaminated with bacteria, so washing is an important step in the juicing process.

Line your juicer's pulp basket. If you have a juicer with a pulp basket, line it with a plastic bag so that cleaning it is easy. Look for biodegradable bags that you can throw straight into the compost along with your pulp. Remember that pulp can also be used to boost the nutritional and fibre content of certain recipes. Visit page 31 and www.rebootwithjoe.com for more tips on what to do with your pulp, from composting to making broth and baking muffins.

Cut or tear produce to size. It must be able to fit through the juicer's feeder tube, so cut any produce that might be too large to fit. Remember, this is best done just before juicing.

Feed produce through the juicer's feeder tube. If your machine has more than one speed, don't forget to downshift from high to low for soft fruits (the instruction manual should be able to guide you about speeds). Usually, hard produce, such as apples and beetroot (beets) are juiced on high, while soft ones, such as spinach and cabbage, are set to low.

Re-juice your pulp. Once produce has been passed through the juicer, check to see if the pulp is still damp. If it is, pass it back through the juicer and you'll be able to get more juice from it.

Drink up. At this point, you should have a fresh juice ready to drink. If you prefer it cold, pour over ice, but whatever the case, drink it as soon as possible because once it's juiced, it starts to lose its nutritional value. If stored properly (see p. 13) it can last 2–3 days, but remember that there are no preservatives in fresh juice (which is why we love it), so it can quickly go bad.

Now it's time to clean your juicer. Carefully scrub the machine with warm water and soap and place on a drying mat. If it's dishwasher friendly (check the manual), you'll have an even easier clean.

EAT THE RAINBOW

Eat the rainbow sounds like a fun way to eat, but what does it mean? It means over the course of a day, mix it up, eat a variety of colours, and over a week eat a variety of different whites, yellows, oranges, reds, greens and purples (the juicing rainbow). Orange fruits and vegetables, such as carrots and oranges, get their vibrant hue from beta carotene and an abundance of antioxidants, vitamins, fibre and phytonutrients that are good for your skin, eyes and heart. They also contain high amounts of vitamin A that help protect your body against free radicals, and vitamin C which helps boost the immune system. Red produce like beetroots (beets) and cherries are high in anthocyanins (antioxidants) and bring a host of vitamins, minerals and other antioxidants that can help your body fight off disease and stay healthy. Beetroot in particular contains a nutrient called betalain, which has been shown to provide antioxidants, help promote anti-inflammation and is excellent for pre-workouts because it helps bring more oxygen to the blood. Leafy greens, my favourites, are super high in chlorophyll and give me the energy to keep going forever! Not to mention the extreme concentration of phytonutrients, vitamins and minerals needed to function properly. Now think about it, if you combine all of these colours you'll help your body stay strong and healthy.

Tips for storing juice

Place in an airtight container. Glass is ideal, but BPA-free plastic works too. (Some authorities, such as the US Food and Drug Administration, advise against Biphenol-A (BPA), an industrial chemical often used in the manufacture of plastic. Some research studies have linked BPA to breast cancer and diabetes, as well as to hyperactivity, aggression and depression in children.[2])

Fill the container to the top. This will prevent oxygen from getting in, which can deplete the nutrients.

Keep for 2–3 days in the fridge (72 hours is the maximum time suggested). If you are travelling, take your juice in a cooler. Do not use an aluminium Thermos or vacuum flask as metal can react with the juice.

Freeze it for up to 10 days. If you will not be drinking the juice within 48 hours, it is best to freeze it immediately. Thaw in the refrigerator when needed. Make sure you drink the whole amount within 10 days of freezing.

To peel or not to peel?

I love lemon peel in my juice but have to admit I seem to be a bit unusual. If I am making my Mean Green for a first-time juicer, I leave out the peel as I don't want to scare anyone away from juicing. But in a citrus fruit there are over 60 flavonoids, with the highest concentration being within the peel. (Flavonoids are substances found in plants, many of which are responsible for the yellow, orange and red pigmentation. And they're really good for you.) The 'pith' – the white part right under the peel on a citrus fruit – also contains lots of nutrients. So if you really can't handle the peel in your juice, try to leave on the pith. In this case, I recommend cutting off the peel so you can leave on more of the pith.

In general, the outer layers of fruits and vegetables often provide more nutrition than the food they protect. Gram for gram, citrus peels also contain higher levels of many minerals and vitamins, such as vitamin C and dietary fibre, than the fruit's flesh. For example, 1 tablespoon of lemon peel contains double the amount of vitamin C and triple the amount of fibre than 1 wedge of lemon without the peel, according to the United States Department of Agriculture (USDA) database. So for most fruits and vegetables, leave the peels on. Here are a few other peels and skins you might not think you could juice – but you can:

Watermelon

Watermelon rind is excellent for juicing – it is lower in sugar content than the flesh, and higher in potassium and dietary fibre. If you are throwing away the rind, not only are you discarding about 40 per cent of the fresh weight of the watermelon, but you are also losing a potent source of citrulline. Citrulline is an amino acid that is converted to arginine in the body. Arginine increases blood flow, decreasing blood pressure and improving overall cardiovascular health.

As with citrus fruits, the white part of the rind is full of nutrients. If the whole rind is too much flavour for your juice, try leaving some of the white rind on the watermelon flesh when you cut it up.

Mangoes

Don't skin mangoes before you juice them, this part of the fruit contains a significant amount of antioxidants and healthful compounds that are only found in small amounts in the mango pulp. Mangiferin, a phytonutrient found in large amounts in the skin, is a powerful antioxidant. Mangiferin may be helpful in protecting against skin cancer and this UV-protectant ability is valued in the cosmetics industry. Of course, don't skip the SPF!

Beware of mango itch! While mango skin is edible, be careful because it can cause an allergic reaction in some people. Known as 'mango itch' in Hawaii, the sap of the mango tree and mango skin contain urushiol, the same compound responsible for the itchy skin rash seen in poison ivy and poison oak. People who are sensitive to poison ivy and poison oak may also be sensitive to the urushiol in mangoes and should avoid eating or juicing the skin.

Apples

Apples might be a little more obvious to you since it's common to eat them with the skins on, but you'd be surprised to know that many people prefer to eat apples after peeling off the skin. If you're one of them, you might want to reconsider because the majority of the apple's nutrients are found in the peel. The peel is loaded with vitamins A and C, and heaps of minerals like calcium, potassium and iron. Let's not forget about the fibre! About two-thirds of an apple's fibre, both soluble and insoluble, exists in its peel.

With any peels, if you do juice or eat them, it is best to use organic products, because the peel is where pesticide residue can be concentrated. Whether you purchase organic or not, be sure to wash your fruits well before juicing, blending or eating them. Try a home remedy wash with vinegar, lemon, bicarbonate of soda (baking soda) and water to help remove pesticide residue.

Don't want to juice them? Eat them!

● **Citrus peels** – Zest or grate citrus peels to infuse their essence within smoothies and baked goods. Grated or finely chopped peels also add a bright flavouring to savoury dishes and sauces.

● **Mango peels** – Mangoes can be eaten raw with their skin on, though some people may not like the texture or feel the taste is bitter. If you find that to be the case, cut up the mango with its skin and blend in a high-powered blender, mixing with other fruits and vegetables. Choose some of the thinner-skinned varieties and make sure the fruit is ripe, as that is when the skin is at its thinnest. Mango skin can be pickled or sun- or oven-dried to make a crunchy chip.

● **Watermelon rind** – Instead of throwing the white rind away, leave some of it attached when you cut up the watermelon flesh. You can juice the watermelon this way, or add it to smoothies. If you find the result a little bitter, the addition of sweet fruits and/or spices such as fresh ginger will offset this. Pickled watermelon rind is also a classic Southern alternative to pickles in the US.

● **Apples** – Rinse well before eating then bite right into it or slice it up in smaller pieces and top with your favourite nut butter for a heartier snack.

● **Leek leaves** – Did you know that leeks are one of the most iron-rich plant foods – they contain more iron than spinach! I've always thrown away the leaf – the dark green part of the leek at the top – in favour of the white and light green parts (no, it's not a peel, it's something we typically throw away and shouldn't!). I was always told that the dark green parts weren't edible. Boy, was I told wrong. While the green leaves are thicker than the shaft of the leek, they only need a little time to cook. The secret is to slice them fairly thinly, in rounds or strips. Slicing diagonally is another helpful trick. Braise them in a little stock, or sauté them in a little oil over medium heat until lightly browned and use as a garnish. Chop them up and add them to your vegetables when making stocks. If you blanch them first (to make them malleable), you can also use the leaves to roll with tofu, fish or other protein, infusing it with a mild oniony flavour.

Juicing produce preparation guide

Not sure what to do with those fruits, veggies and spices before you put them in your juicer? Here's a list of how to prepare the most commonly used ingredients. Once you've gained confidence by making the juices in this book, get creative and start experimenting with your own combinations. You can also find more juice recipes at www.rebootwithjoe.com/recipes.

VEGETABLES	HOW TO PREPARE
Asparagus	Rinse the spears (stalks) carefully and push through juicer, bottom first.
Aubergine (eggplant)	I've never juiced aubergine and I don't think I ever will. In my opinion, it's best for eating.
Beetroot (beets)	Peel if you wish to avoid the 'earthy' taste that many people dislike, and cut to fit your juicer. Juice their greens too.
Beets	*see* Beetroot
Bell peppers	*see* Sweet (bell) peppers
Broccoli	After rinsing, juice all parts.
Butterhead lettuce	Rinse leaves individually, checking for dirt and sand. No need to remove the stems. Roll the leaves up and feed into the juicer, following each batch with a harder fruit or vegetable, such as apple, celery or cucumber, to help them pass through.
Cabbage, green and red	The cabbage head should be firm with crisp leaves. Cut into quarters, or smaller if necessary, to fit into the juicer's feeder tube.
Capsicums	*see* Sweet (bell) peppers
Carrots	Rinse thoroughly before passing through the juicer. No need to peel them or discard the greens.
Celeriac (celery root)	Wash carefully, as grit can get stuck in the nooks and crannies. As with beetroot, if you don't like an earthy taste, peel the celeriac first. Cut to fit your juicer.
Celery	Rinse thoroughly and pass the entire celery stalk, including leaves, through the juicer.
Celery root	*see* Celeriac
Chard (silverbeet)	Rinse leaves individually, checking for dirt and sand. No need to remove the stems. Roll up and feed into the juicer, following each batch with a harder fruit or vegetable, such as apple, celery or cucumber, to help them pass through.

VEGETABLES	HOW TO PREPARE
Collard greens (spring greens can be used in UK)	Wash the leaves. No need to remove the stems. Roll up and feed into the juicer, following each batch with a harder fruit or vegetable, such as apple, celery or cucumber, to help them pass through.
Cos lettuce	*see* Romaine
Courgettes (zucchini)	Scrub and cut off stem, but leave the rounded end on. These are great for pushing through leafy greens.
Cucumbers	Cut in half. No need to peel.
Dandelions	Wash the leaves. No need to remove the stems. Roll up and feed into the juicer, following each batch with a harder fruit or vegetable, such as apple, celery or cucumber, to help them pass through. These leaves have some bite to them, so use sparingly, or soften the flavour with a sweet and juicy fruit, such as pineapple.
Eggplant	*see* Aubergine
Fennel	Rinse and chop the bulb to fit through the juicer. You can also juice the fronds for extra nutrients. Fennel has a light aniseed flavour, which reminds me of liquorice.
Jicama (yam bean, Mexican turnip – not available in UK)	Wash and slice, but don't peel. The resulting juice will contain nutrients that were near the skin even after the skin has been pulped away.
Kai choi	*see* Mustard greens
Kale (Tuscan cabbage)	Use any kind – lacinato, red, green, purple, curly, etc. Wash the leaves, then roll up 3–4 at a time and feed into the juicer, following each batch with a harder fruit or vegetable, such as apple, celery or cucumber, to help them pass through.
Kohlrabi	Both leaves and bulb can be juiced, but the flavour (similar to broccoli) is strong, so aim for a juice to contain no more than 25 per cent kohlrabi.

VEGETABLES	HOW TO PREPARE
Leeks	Trim off the woody base, then slice both green and white parts in half lengthways. Gently separate the layers and rinse between them.
Mustard greens (kai choi)	Use just a small amount as they have a strong flavour that will literally warm your insides. Wash the leaves. No need to remove the stems. Roll up and feed into the juicer, following each batch with a harder fruit or vegetable, such as apple, celery or cucumber, to help them pass through.
Onions	Go easy on these, as they can give your juices a super-strong flavour. Some people prefer not to juice them at all, especially if raw onion upsets their stomach. Peel off the papery skin, then chop to fit your juicer. Add to your juice a little at a time, tasting as you go, and adding more if you like it.
Parsnips	Rinse thoroughly before passing through the juicer. No need to peel them. You might need to slice large ones in half lengthways. These can be used to help push leafy greens through your juicer.
Pumpkin	*see* Squashes
Radishes	Leave the root and stem on, but discard the leaves if they have any. Rinse and run through your juicer. Watch out! These can spice up your juice in a flash, so add small amounts at a time. If you're feeling cold, adding these to your juice will warm you right up.
Romaine (cos) lettuce	Rinse leaves individually, checking for dirt and sand. No need to remove the stems. Roll up and feed into the juicer, following each batch with a harder fruit or vegetable, such as apple, celery or cucumber, to help them pass through.

VEGETABLES	HOW TO PREPARE
Scallions	*see* Spring onions
Silverbeet	*see* Chard
Spinach	Wash well – some bunches can have a lot of grit on them. No need to remove the stems. Roll up and feed into the juicer, following each batch with a harder fruit or vegetable, such as apple, celery or cucumber, to help them pass through.
Spring onions (scallions)	Just rinse and juice. No need to remove the roots or dark green parts because you can juice it all. These have a strong flavour, like onions, so start small.
Squashes (including pumpkin)	Remove the stem and scrub the skin. If the skin is really tough and thick, you might want to peel it. Otherwise, slice and keep the seeds in (they provide extra cancer-fighting chemicals), and pass through the juicer.
Sugarsnap peas	Rinse and run through juicer. These don't have a very high water content, so they don't yield a lot of juice. Try juicing them with carrots.
Sweet (bell) peppers (capsicums)	Rinse, then remove the stem – it's fine to retain the seeds. Cut to size and juice.
Sweet potatoes	Scrub and cut into chunks. Combine them with peaches, pears and/or apples and you'll have a delicious dessert juice.
Tomatoes	Wash, then remove the stem and any leaves. Keep the seeds. If large, slice to fit your juicer. Fresh tomato juice is worlds away from the canned stuff.
Turnips	Scrub and chop in chunks to fit your juicer. A great addition to a juice for cooler weather.
Tuscan cabbage	*see* Kale

VEGETABLES	HOW TO PREPARE
Wheatgrass	Some juicers are better at doing wheatgrass than others. If you're preparing just a small amount, any kind of juicer should be able to handle it. Rinse the wheatgrass, twist or roll into a ball, and push it through the machine with something juicy and firm, such as apples. Adding wheatgrass will give a strong green flavour to the juice, and provide lots of great chlorophyll energy.
Zucchini	*see* Courgettes

FRUITS	HOW TO PREPARE
Apples	Core and remove the seeds before pushing through the juicer.
Apricots	Rinse and slice in half to remove the stone (pit).
Avocados	Peel and remove the stone (pit) – easily lifted out with a spoon. The flesh is great for thickening juices in a blender, but never put an avocado in a juicer.
Bananas	Peel, but never juice bananas. Like avocados, they are great for thickening juices in a blender.
Blackberries	Rinse in a strainer. They don't keep well after being rinsed, so wash them the day you plan to juice them.
Blueberries	Rinse in a strainer.
Cactus pears	*see* Prickly pears
Chayotes (chokos)	Wash and chop to size. No need to peel or remove seed.
Cherries	Remove stalks, then rinse the fruit. Use a small paring knife to remove the hard stones (pits) before juicing.
Chokos	*see* Chayotes
Cranberries	Rinse and pass through the juicer. Make sure you juice them with something sweet because these will taste really tart, not like ready-made cranberry juice.
Grapefruit	Peel thinly, keeping as much of the white pith on the fruit as possible (it contains nutrients that help the body to absorb the vitamin C and amazing antioxidants found in citrus fruits). Cut to fit the juicer and remove the seeds. If you have a centrifugal juicer, you can keep the seeds in: they contain excellent nutrients too.
Grapes	Wash the grapes and remove from their stems. Pass them through the juicer. Experiment with different colours because they yield different flavours.

FRUITS	HOW TO PREPARE
Kiwi fruit	Peel and run through the juicer, seeds and all.
Kumquats	Rinse, no need to peel.
Lemons	Peel thinly, keeping as much of the white pith on the fruit as possible (it contains nutrients that help the body to absorb the vitamin C and amazing antioxidants found in citrus fruits). Cut to fit the juicer and remove the seeds. If you have a centrifugal juicer, you can keep the seeds in: they contain excellent nutrients too.
Limes	Peel thinly, keeping as much of the white pith on the fruit as possible (it contains nutrients that help the body to absorb the vitamin C and amazing antioxidants found in citrus fruits). Cut to fit the juicer and remove the seeds. If you have a centrifugal juicer, you can keep the seeds in: they contain excellent nutrients too.
Mangos	Peel and cut spears of flesh by making angled incisions down to the large, flat stone (pit) in the middle. Makes a great tropical juice when mixed with pineapple. Also imparts a great creamy texture.
Melons	Cantaloupe (rockmelon) has orange flesh, which should be cut into wedges, then peeled and deseeded before juicing. Other types of melon, e.g. Charentais, Galia, Honeydew, can be juiced with their seeds.
Oranges	Peel thinly, keeping as much of the white pith on the fruit as possible (it contains nutrients that help the body to absorb the vitamin C and amazing antioxidants found in citrus fruits). Cut to fit the juicer and remove the seeds. If you have a centrifugal juicer, you can keep the seeds in: they contain excellent nutrients too.
Papaya	Cut in half and peel off the skin. The seeds can be juiced with the flesh.

FRUITS	HOW TO PREPARE
Peaches	Cut in half to remove the stone (pit), then pass through the juicer.
Pears	Remove the stem, then wash and juice whole. Slice to fit your juicer if necessary.
Pineapples	The heavier the pineapple, the riper it is. Grab hold of the top and twist off (you might want to wear gloves for this). Slice into quarters, cut out the woody core, then peel off the skin, and juice.
Plums	Wash and slice in half to remove the stone (pit). I love experimenting with different types of plums – there are so many. They give your juice a gorgeous colour with an antioxidant punch.
Pomegranates	I have a great trick for dealing with this fruit. Fill a bowl with water, then slice the pomegranate in half, keeping the halves together. Submerge it in the water, then break it apart – this prevents the juice from squirting everywhere. Keeping it in the water, break the pomegranate into chunks and tease the seeds out. The white parts and skin will float and the seeds will sink. Discard all the skin and white parts from the surface of the water and use a slotted spoon to lift out the seeds. Juice them in their entirety.
Prickly pears (cactus pears)	Wear gloves when handling these if the spines have not already been removed. Peel and cut to size if necessary.
Raspberries	Rinse and juice. I love to add a little bit of lemon to a juice made with raspberries, or combine them with fresh peaches for a peach melba juice.
Strawberries	As these have a powerful flavour when juiced, I like to mix them with other berries, or maybe one or two other fruits. Just rinse, discard the leafy bits and pop right in the juicer.

FRUITS	HOW TO PREPARE
Tangerines	Peel thinly, keeping as much of the white pith on the fruit as possible (it contains nutrients that help the body to absorb the vitamin C and amazing antioxidants found in citrus fruits). Cut to fit the juicer and remove the seeds. If you have a centrifugal juicer, you can keep the seeds in: they contain excellent nutrients too.
Watermelon	Makes an amazingly refreshing juice, especially in hot weather. Simply cut into wedges and juice the rind, flesh and seeds.

HERBS AND SPICES	HOW TO PREPARE
Basil	Wash carefully, swishing the bunch in a bowl of cold water if it seems very gritty. Tear the leaves off the stems, roll them up and feed into the juicer, pushing them through with firmer produce.
Chilli peppers (jalapeño)	Discard the stem. Wash and juice. Chillies are pretty spicy, so use with care. If you want a milder flavour, discard the seeds.
Chinese five-spice powder	Don't put this through the juicer – just sprinkle into your juice.
Coriander (cilantro)	Wash thoroughly and juice both stems and leaves.
Cinnamon, ground	Don't put this through the juicer. Sprinkle it on juices, such as apple, pear or sweet potato.
Dill	Rinse and pull the delicate fronds off the stem to juice them.
Garlic	The flavour is strong and so are the benefits – too many to list here, but trust me, garlic is a wonderfood. Use fresh garlic and peel before running through the juicer. Start with a small amount and taste your juice before adding more.
Ginger	Cut off the size piece you need for your juice, then use a spoon to peel off the skin off (I find this just as effective as using a knife). Ginger doesn't produce much juice, but it does add a distinctive flavour, so be careful not to go overboard.
Mint	Wash thoroughly and juice only the leaves. The flavour is great with grapes, pineapple, strawberries and watermelon.

HERBS AND SPICES	HOW TO PREPARE
Parsley	Wash well, swishing the whole bunch in water if very gritty. Tear the leaves off the stems, roll them up and feed into the juicer, pushing them through with firmer produce.
Tarragon	Gives a slight flavour of aniseed to vegetable juices. Wash and tear the leaves off their woody stems before juicing.

Substitution guide for juice ingredients

PRODUCE	ALTERNATIVES
Apple	Blackberries, cherries, grapes, honeydew melon, mango, peach, pear, pineapple
Arugula	*see* Rocket
Asparagus	Broccoli stalks, green beans
Basil	Coriander (cilantro), mint, parsley
Beetroot	Golden beetroot, radish, red cabbage, tomato
Beet greens	Collard greens, dandelion greens, kale (Tuscan cabbage), mustard greens, rocket (arugula), spinach, spring greens, watercress
Blueberries	Blackberries, cherries, raspberries, strawberries
Broccoli florets	Cauliflower, green cabbage
Broccoli stalks	Asparagus, celery, cucumber, cauliflower
Butternut squash	*see* Squash, winter
Cabbage, green	Kale (Tuscan cabbage), red/purple cabbage, rocket (arugula), sweet green (bell) pepper, watercress
Cabbage, red/purple	Broccoli, cauliflower, green cabbage, radicchio, radish, tomato
Cantaloupe melon	Honeydew melon, mango, papaya, peach
Capsicum	*see* Sweet green/red/yellow (bell) pepper
Carrot	Butternut squash (pumpkin), parsnip, sweet potato
Celeriac (celery root)	Celery, jicama (yam bean), kohlrabi, turnip
Celery	Cucumber, jicama (yam bean, Mexican turnip), courgette (zucchini)
Celery root	*see* Celeriac

PRODUCE	ALTERNATIVES
Chard	Beet greens, collard greens, green cabbage, kale (Tuscan cabbage), mustard greens, rocket (arugula), romaine lettuce, spinach, spring greens, watercress
Cherries	Blackberries, blueberries, raspberries, strawberries
Chilli pepper (jalapeño)	Serrano pepper, sweet yellow or green (bell) pepper
Cilantro	*see* Coriander
Collard greens	Beet greens, chard, green cabbage, kale (Tuscan cabbage), mustard greens, rocket (arugula), romaine lettuce, spinach, spring greens, watercress
Coriander	Basil, mint, parsley
Cos lettuce	*see* Romaine
Courgette (zucchini)	Celery, cucumber, summer squash
Cranberries	Blackberries, cherries, raspberries
Cucumber	Celery, jicama (yam bean), courgette (zucchini)
Dandelion greens	Beet greens, collard greens, kale (Tuscan cabbage), mustard greens, spring greens
Fennel	Celery root, jicama (yam bean), kohlrabi
Garlic	Shallots, spring onions (scallions)
Ginger	Lemon, lime
Grapefruit	Blood orange, clementine, orange, star fruit, tangerine
Grapes	Apple, honeydew melon
Honeydew melon	Apple, cantaloupe, grapes
Jalapeño	*see* Chilli pepper
Kai choi	*see* Mustard greens
Kale (Tuscan cabbage)	Beet greens, chard, collard greens, green cabbage, mustard greens, rocket (arugula), spinach, spring greens, watercress
Kiwi fruit	Lime, mango, orange, tangerine

PRODUCE	ALTERNATIVES
Kumquat	Tangerine, clementine, grapefruit, orange
Leek	Garlic, onion, shallot
Lemon	Clementine, ginger, lime, orange, tangerine
Lime	Clementine, ginger, lemon, orange, tangerine
Mango	Kiwi fruit, orange, papaya, pineapple
Mint	Basil, coriander (cilantro), ginger
Onion	Garlic, leek, shallot
Orange	Clementine, grapefruit, kiwi fruit, lemon, lime, mango, papaya, tangerine
Oregano	Sage
Parsley	Rocket (arugula), basil, coriander (cilantro), kale (Tuscan cabbage)
Parsnip	Celeriac, sweet potato, turnip, winter squash
Peach	Apple, orange, pear, plum
Pear	Apple, celeriac, peach, plum
Pineapple	Grapefruit, mango, orange, pomegranate
Pomegranate	Cherries, pineapple, strawberries
Pumpkin	*see* Squash, winter
Radish	Beetroot, red/purple cabbage, sweet red (bell) pepper, tomato
Raspberries	Blackberries, blueberries, cherries, strawberries
Rocket (arugula)	Beetroot greens, chard, collard greens, dandelion greens, green cabbage, kale (Tuscan cabbage), parsley, spinach, spring greens, watercress
Rockmelon	*see* Cantaloupe
Romaine lettuce	Butterhead lettuce, green or red leaf lettuce, radicchio
Scallion	*see* Spring onion
Shallot	Garlic, onion, spring onion (scallion)
Silverbeet	*see* Chard

PRODUCE	ALTERNATIVES
Spinach	Beet greens, chard, collard greens, dandelion greens, kale (Tuscan cabbage), mustard greens, romaine lettuce, spring greens
Spring onion (scallion)	Garlic, onion, shallot
Squash, summer	Cucumber, courgette (zucchini)
Squash, winter	Carrot, parsnip, sweet potato
Strawberries	Blackberries, cherries, raspberries
Sweet green (bell) pepper	Green cabbage, sweet red or yellow (bell) pepper
Sweet potato	Butternut squash, carrot, parsnip
Sweet red (bell) pepper	Radish, sweet yellow or green (bell) pepper, tomato, watermelon
Sweet yellow (bell) pepper	Sweet green or red (bell) pepper, yellow tomato, pineapple
Tangerine	Grapefruit, lemon, orange
Tomato	Radish, red/purple cabbage, sweet red (bell) pepper, watermelon
Tuscan cabbage	*see* Kale
Watermelon	Cantaloupe, grapefruit, honeydew melon
Zucchini	*see* Courgette

Let's talk about pulp

'I love juicing but hate wasting all that pulp!' This is a common complaint I hear about juicing. The good news is there are plenty of uses for pulp. I asked our Reboot community what they do with it, and they came back with a whole book of ideas. Here are a few of my favourite ones. We've also included a selection of pulp recipes in the recipes chapter.

1 Make your own veggie broth! (See p. 229.)

2 Add to your favourite vegetarian burger recipe. It adds flavour, texture, moisture and nutrition (see p. 233).

3 Mix it in with your next smoothie for additional fibre.

4 Compost it and add it to your garden.

5 Make an Italian favourite, spaghetti and meatballs, into a nutrient-rich dish by using pulp to make Vegetarian Meatballs (see p. 235).

6 If you don't have time to use the pulp immediately, place it in resealable bags and freeze it until you need it.

7 Feed it to your furry friends! Add a little leftover kale pulp to your dog's food bowl and watch them scarf it down. You can also make nutritious dog treats (see p. 241).

8 If you have a hard time getting your kids to eat their vegetables, try adding the pulp to sauces, soups and other dinner ingredients – they'll never know it's in there.

9 Make Banana Carrot and Courgette (Zucchini) Muffins (see p. 233).

10 Raise your own chickens? Feed it to them!

11 Stir it right into your soups for added flavour and, of course, more nutrients.

12 Make gluten-free, raw Rosemary Carrot Flax Crackers (see p. 235).

13 Use as a spread on sandwiches and crackers.

14 Add it to your favourite stir fry or even omelette or frittata recipe.

15 Freeze the pulp after juicing ginger root and use it as a topical anaesthetic for sore muscles and bruises.

16 Make a homemade face scrub. Anything from cucumbers, carrots, lemons, oranges, parsley, kale, radish, etc. can be applied directly to your face. You can also mix in a bit of honey or oatmeal to help it stick.

17 Sprinkle it on a salad for added benefits.

18 Try it as an indoor plant fertiliser.

19 Use pulp from apples to make apple sauce. Add a little ground cinnamon and a pinch of coconut sugar over a frying pan and warm until it reaches a nice consistency.

20 Enjoy it as its own salad. Think apple, carrot and ginger pulp with chopped pineapple and coconut flakes!

21 If you have a dehydrator, dehydrate for a crunchy salad topping.

22 Mix leafy green pulp into your favourite healthy whole grain like brown rice, quinoa and millet.

How to get the most nutritious delicious produce

I'm asked quite often which juicer produces the most nutritious juice, but the truth is, there are multiple factors that affect the nutritional quality of your juice (and your food) – and it's not down to the juicer. The most important factor may be the actual produce. Not all cobs of corn or tomatoes are created equal. One of the twenty-first-century triumphs of agriculture is that we have been able to increase crop yields to feed an ever-expanding global population. But the cost of higher yields is decreased nutritional quality in the foods we are growing. Some studies show that today's produce contains 10–25 per cent less iron, zinc, protein, calcium, vitamins and other nutrients than historic crops.[3]

Other studies show that organic produce may

actually be more nutritious than conventional produce. It seems that the pesticides and fertilisers that are meant to protect plants and create higher yields actually weaken their nutritional quality. A recent study found that organic tomatoes have double the amounts of antioxidants compared to conventional tomatoes.[4] And did you know that often the more bitter fruits and vegetables have higher concentrations of phytonutrients?[5]

There are other things that affect the nutritional density of all produce, whether it is high-yield, heirloom, conventional, sweet or bitter, and that is exposure to oxygen, light and heat. As soon as produce is picked, it starts to lose its nutritional quality. Why is that? Because as soon as it is picked, nutrients begin to oxidize into the air. The more extreme the light and heat exposure, the more rapid the nutrient loss. Leafy greens with a large surface area and no hard protective covering cannot be stored as long as other fruits and vegetables and lose their nutritional density relatively rapidly. Peels on citrus fruit and the rinds on melons protect their fruits from light and oxygen, which is why oranges and cantaloupes last longer if you don't cut them. Once exposed to oxygen, bacteria in the air also start to work, helping produce decay. Refrigerating food slows down the bacterial action, so it takes food longer to spoil. Freezing food stops the bacterial process (frozen bacteria are inactive) and some fruits and vegetables can be frozen up to a year without losing their nutritional density.

For some fruits and vegetables, the cooking process – heating food to 46°C/115°F or higher – can also decrease their nutritional density. However this is not true for tomatoes: cooking tomatoes actually increases their concentration of lycopene, which has important cancer-fighting properties.

This is why I'm a fan of HPP bottled juices – HPP bottled juice is produced using high pressure to pasteurise the juice, not heat, so fewer nutrients are lost in the bottling process. Making your own juice is still best but HPP juices are a great option when you can't make your own. I know what you're thinking, 'Joe, isn't a raw food diet best then?' Well I'm not someone who can live on raw food! While I eat a lot of raw foods I also enjoy soups and vegetarian mains (and occasional ice cream and meat!). And I know that cooked fruits and veggies have an amazing amount of nutrition. For some the cooking process actually increases the absorption of nutrients. That's why you can enjoy cooked vegetables during the eating portion of your Reboot.

What does this mean for you? The bottom line is, if you can, buy local (food is generally fresher if it hasn't travelled halfway across the world), look for heirloom varieties, buy organic, and use your produce as quickly as possible after you buy it – don't shove it in the fridge for a week. And know that frozen produce may not only be cheaper but might also be more nutritious than the same item out of season in the produce aisle. If you can't follow any of these suggestions, don't worry. I'll take conventionally grown carrots that were shipped across the country and have sat in my fridge for seven days over 90 per cent of the items on supermarket shelves.

As far as the most nutritious juicer goes, I don't think it matters much. There are no juicers on the market that heat up produce enough to kill nutrients. (My favourite, the Breville Juice Fountain Plus, heats up the produce one degree during the spinning process.) Use the juicer that works best for you and don't worry about which is most nutritious. Juice is nutritious – just juice on!

Juicing, blending, what's the difference?

They're both great, but they are *really* different and it's important to understand why. When you blend, everything goes into a machine, you hit the "whiz" button and then everything that went into the machine is poured out into your glass. You won't see the blueberries, chunks of apples or kale leaves anymore... but they're all in the glass. It's the same calories and nutrition as eating them whole – just faster and more delicious.

When you juice, everything goes into the machine, but the liquid is separated from the solids. You will have a glass of juice and a separate container of pulp. If you don't have leftover pulp, you're not juicing. It's almost three quarters of the nutrition as eating the ingredients whole, but in a form that allows your body to quickly absorb the nutrients and gives your digestive system a break.

So which one is better? They're both great for you! When you juice, you are removing the insoluble fibre but you are retaining 65 to 70 per cent of the nutrients that are in the produce. And without fibre to slow down your digestion, your body rapidly absorbs the nutrients. Try eating 70 per cent of the produce that goes into my Mean Green. And then do that five times a day. That's a lot of eating! That's why on a Reboot we recommend juicing. By juicing you are supercharging your body with nutrients. We've noticed weight loss tends to be faster when juicing too. And after a lot of practice, I can tell you that there are some vegetables – beetroot, sweet potatoes, squash – that I think are just much better juiced.

When you blend, you are retaining the insoluble fibre. And yes, fibre is good for you. It helps maintain healthy bowels, lowers cholesterol levels and slows the absorption of sugar – which is particularly important for diabetics. This is why our Reboot plans call for juices that are primarily made from vegetables (80 per cent veggies to 20 per cent fruit). Not only do they provide an important variety of nutrients, they are much lower in sugar. And if your post-Reboot diet is high in plant foods (which I hope it is!), you will be getting lots of fibre.

When I'm not Rebooting, I like both juices and smoothies. I will make a Mean Green juice almost every day since it is such a delicious and efficient way to fuel my body. And sometimes I feel like having a Green Monkey with almond milk, bananas and almond butter – ingredients you can't juice.

SHOPPING & COOKING

Produce shopping

When fruits and veggies become a bigger part of your life, so do trips to the farmers' market and grocery store. No more sitting in line at the drive-thru for your fast food! This means you have to spend more time preparing to shop, know what to look for while you are there, and learn the best way to store the beautiful fresh produce when you get home. Once you get the hang of it, it's all pretty simple. Follow these guidelines to make your next visit to the farmers' market or grocery store quick, easy and affordable. Happy shopping!

Before shopping for produce

1 **Make your shopping list:** Go prepared with a detailed list so you know exactly what you need. Not only

will this make your trip faster but it will also help you avoid succumbing to any unhealthy temptations.

2 **Research seasonal produce:** Produce that's currently in season will be easier to find and will likely be the best price. Berries in the summer are half the price that they are in the winter.

3 **Eat a small snack at home:** Never go shopping for food when you are hungry. An empty stomach in the grocery store might lead to selecting unhealthy food choices.

4 **Bring reusable grocery bags:** Save paper and plastic and use your own bags. It's a great way to carry home (or to your car) your purchases versus 10 plastic bags hanging from your arms, and it cuts down on waste.

5 **Bring the whole family:** Make it a family outing. It's a great opportunity to teach your children about healthy eating. They also make great shoppers when selecting new fruits and veggies to try!

At the market or grocery store

1 **Bright is best:** Always select the fruits and vegetables that are brightest in colour. If something is greying and discoloured, it indicates spoiling. (Note: Avocados are the exception to this rule. Most bright green avocados are not ripe yet, so look for darker skin with a lightly firm touch.)

2 No wrinkles: Wrinkled, bruised and cracked produce can indicate the produce is spoiling. This isn't always the case, though, and much of your produce can still be used, especially in a smoothie or a juice. But you be the judge – if it doesn't look like it typically should be used, don't buy it.

3 In season: Always try to shop in season! Seasonal produce is typically the cheapest and ripest. If you're shopping at a farmers' market, you'll likely only have seasonal options so it will be easy.

4 Fresh smell: Our sense of smell can be the best indicator of freshness. If it smells bad, put it down.

5 No bags: We know this isn't always easy, but when possible don't buy any produce that is sold in plastic bags, unless it is coming directly from a farmer! And even when you pick up loose apples off the shelf in a grocery store, you don't need to put them in a plastic bag, just throw them right in your trolley or your reusable grocery bag.

6 Size matters: Certain produce, like grapes and bananas, are often sold in plastic bags, but remember you don't always need to buy the whole bag! You can separate a bunch of bananas or a bundle of grapes and take only what you need.

7 Dirt is your friend: If the produce is fresh off the farm it doesn't always look perfect. It may have a little dirt on it, it might not be perfectly shaped, but you will know it is fresh and nutrient-rich.

8 The price is right: Pay attention to the posted price. Is it per-pound or per-unit? If priced by unit, then go for the heaviest and biggest one you can find! If priced by weight, then grabbing a smaller amount consistent with how much you plan to use will save you some money.

9 Prioritise organic: Prioritise and buy the organic items that are considered the 'Dirty Dozen' by the Environmental Working Group in the US (listed on page 50). The 'Clean Fifteen' (page 51) do not contain as many pesticides, so if you are watching your wallet you can skip these in the organic aisle.

10 Frequent the freezer section: Don't forget the freezer section, where frozen organic fruits and vegetables are always available. They last longer than fresh produce, they are high in nutrients and they often go on sale.

Storing produce at home

1 Determine the best location: In the fridge or on the counter? If you do not know what produce you should refrigerate and what you should store at room temperature, notice how the grocery store stores it; if they keep something at room temperature, then so should you. If you're at the farmers' market, ask them!

2 Know your fruits: If storing in the fridge, place fruits in the produce drawer. Keep fruits that produce ethylene, such as apples, cantaloupe, honeydew melons, tomatoes and bananas, away from other fruits and vegetables. Store fruits on the countertop with care. Keep fruits in large baskets or bowls on the countertop uncovered but away from sunlight and direct heat.

3 Know your veggies: When keeping vegetables in the fridge, put them in the crisper to keep them fresh. Vegetables like onions, radishes, carrots, broccoli, cauliflower, leafy greens and squash store best unwashed and in proper storage containers, like BPA-free produce savers. Store herbs by cutting off the ends of the stalks and placing the bunch in a cup of water. Cover the top with a plastic bag.

4 Wait to wash: Don't rinse your fruits and vegetables prior to storing in the refrigerator. Washing these items adds water content, which will increase spoilage rates.

5 Prevent spoiling: If produce you typically store at room temperature starts to brown or become softer, place it in the freezer or fridge! The colder temperature will slow the ripening process. You can also add them to a juice or smoothie immediately so they don't go to waste.

Washing produce

Unwashed fruit and vegetables can be contaminated with bacteria, so it is important to make washing your produce one of the first steps when preparing it for juicing or cooking. Both the National Health Institute in the UK and the Food and Drug Administration (FDA) in the US recommend washing all fruits and vegetables thoroughly in cold, purified water before juicing or eating. If the water is purified it helps avoid harmful pollutants that are often present in tap water.

A few general tips for scrubbing: when washing cabbage or other members of the cruciferous vegetable family, like Brussels sprouts, always remove the outer leaves first since they are generally the most contaminated. For leafy greens, first rinse them under cold running water and then place them in a bowl filled with water to really get them clean. Rinse berries and similar fragile fruits in a colander, while apples, pears and other harder fruits can be scrubbed right under the tap. And don't neglect the produce with outer rinds and peels like pineapple, watermelon, mango and citrus fruits! They need to be washed well too as contaminants on the outer skin may be transferred to the edible parts during peeling or cutting. Root vegetables with thicker skins like sweet potatoes and beetroot (beets) may be scrubbed with a vegetable brush to remove potential bacteria.

If you are concerned about pesticides and/or food-borne bacteria, the following wash is a great natural disinfectant.

Produce wash

8fl oz/250ml/1 cup water
8fl oz/250ml/1 cup white vinegar
1 tbsp bicarbonate of soda (baking soda)
½ lemon

1 Mix the ingredients in a large bowl to allow for the vigorous chemical reaction between the vinegar and bicarb. When the reaction has stopped, pour into a spray bottle.

2 Spray your produce (you can use a scrubbing brush for firm items) and rinse well.

Organic, local or conventional?

That's easy to answer – organic and local! But what if it's the middle of winter, or you don't have organic options, or the organic ones are too expensive? I prefer local whenever possible. Local, seasonal produce is by far the best tasting, and shopping at a farmers' market allows me to support my community and gives me a direct connection with the person growing my produce.

The organic certification process can be costly and time-consuming, so many small-scale local farmers may not be certified organic even though they are not using pesticides. The best way to find out is by asking! Get to know your local farmers; if you are buying directly from the grower you can ask them how their produce is grown.

If you can't find a local option, then look for organic produce. But if organic is out of your budget, don't sweat it. The micronutrients in fruits and vegetables are full of disease-fighting properties. My preference is to eat fruits and vegetables. I prefer conventional to none!

If you can't afford to go completely organic and can only be selective about what organic produce to buy, check out the US-based Environmental Working Groups' list of the most 'dirty' fruits and vegetables, below (for more information visit www.ewg.org/food-news/summary). These are the ones to buy organic if you can. And remember – if you are eating conventional products, peel them before juicing or cooking.

Dirty Dozen Plus

Apples
Celery
Cherry tomatoes
Cucumbers
Grapes
Hot peppers
Kale (Tuscan cabbage)/spring (collard) greens
Nectarines (imported)
Peaches
Potatoes
Spinach
Strawberries
Sweet (bell) peppers (capsicum)
Summer squash

Clean Fifteen

Asparagus
Aubergine (Eggplant)
Avocados
Cabbage
Cantaloupe
Grapefruit
Kiwi
Mangoes
Mushrooms
Onions
Papayas
Peas (frozen)
Pineapples
Sweetcorn
Sweet potatoes

LOCO FOR COCONUT OIL

You'll notice in most of our recipes that require cooking we use coconut oil. Why? Coconut oil is very different from other common cooking oils, like canola and vegetable oils, because it contains a unique composition of 90 per cent saturated fatty acids. This is what gave it such a bad rap for so long, but new studies are emerging that suggest quite the opposite.

Coconut oil is cholesterol-free and contains medium-chain triglycerides ('good fats') and high amounts of lauric acid. The high levels of fatty acids make this oil very resistant to oxidation at high heats, making it ideal for cooking methods that require high temperatures. When oils like olive oil or flax oil are heated above their smoke point, the oil becomes rancid, the chemical structure changes and it will produce blue smoke. Try to use olive oil for fresh salads, so it doesn't need to be heated and you can reap its natural benefits.

If you don't like coconut oil there are other high-quality oils that are excellent for cooking, like avocado oil and macadamia oil. Avocado oil is a great source of mono-unsaturated fatty acids and vitamin E and may even help to boost absorption of carotenoids (a powerful antioxidant) and other nutrients. It naturally has an unusually high smoke point, which means it's good for cooking at medium to high temperatures. Macadamia oil is also among the more heat-stable oils, and, like avocado oil, has a high percentage of monounsaturated fats, which may make it beneficial for heart health and anti-inflammation. It makes for a great oil to cook with at medium to high temperatures, or to use raw on salads or in juices.

Coconut oil doesn't need to be refrigerated. Simply store it on the shelf. At a slightly cool room temperature, it may be solid and on warmer days a liquid. Simply run it under hot water or pop in the microwave if you need it in liquid form. You can sauté with it, or use it in place of oil in almost any recipe. It's great for popping corn or as butter substitute in recipes – try replacing butter with coconut oil in chocolate chip cookies. Sounds crazy, but it's delicious.

You can also use coconut oil in juices or smoothies. In fact, if you plan on Rebooting longer than 15 days we recommend adding 1 teaspoon of coconut oil to one of your juices during the day to help you maintain healthy levels of good-quality fats.

A–Z produce prep for cooking
Reboot-friendly veggies

Acorn squash

Looks like: a acorn-shaped squash with green and orange splashes, should feel firm to the touch with no soft spots.

Prep: Slice in half lengthwise, starting at the stem end, and scoop out the seeds and stringy bits in the middle.

Cook: In the oven: Preheat the oven to 180°C/350°F/ gas 4. Place the two halves of the squash on a baking dish, cut side up, in about 1in/2.5cm of water. Drizzle with coconut oil and sea salt and bake for about 1 hour.

Note: You can eat the skins of acorn squash; when it's cooked well it should have a similar texture to a baked potato skin. It goes great with a bit of maple syrup and cinnamon, if you are craving a little more sweet than savoury.

Artichoke

Looks like: tight green buds – watch out for browning or bruising.

Prep: Use kitchen scissors to snip tough outer leaves and trim the long bottom stem.

Cook: On the stove: heat a bit of coconut oil in a large skillet; add the artichokes and stir for about a minute.

Add 16fl oz/500ml (2 cups) water (or vegetable broth) and 1 teaspoon dried rosemary. Bring to a simmer; cover, reduce the heat and cook for about 15 minutes. **On the grill:** Cut artichokes in half and scoop out the choke (whiskers in the centre). Toss with 1 tablespoon of coconut oil and ½ teaspoon sea salt. Preheat the grill, then place the artichokes over a direct medium heat, turning once or twice, until soft to touch, about 8–10 minutes. **Steam:** Put the artichokes in a large pot with about 2in/5cm of water on the stove over a high heat. Cover and steam until tender, about 15 minutes.

Quick tip: Buy frozen artichoke hearts for a quicker, pre-prepared version of this veggie.

Asparagus

Looks like: green spears, check for freshness by bending, as they should snap when bent.

Prep: Trim the stem ends and rinse.

Cook: In the oven: Preheat the oven to 200°C/400°F/gas 6 and spread the spears over a baking sheet in one layer. Coat with sea salt and coconut oil and cook for about 10 minutes, turning once halfway through. **Steam:** You can quickly prepare asparagus by putting 2in/5cm of water in a pan and placing the asparagus in a steamer basket inside. Cover and steam for about 5 minutes – the spears should be crisp and bright green, just a little more tender. Season with sea salt, pepper, and a drizzle of extra virgin olive oil. **On the**

grill: Make sure the grill rack is oiled, spread out the spears and cook under a medium heat for about 5 minutes, turning occasionally.

Aubergine (Eggplant)

Looks like: a purple bulb with smooth skin, no wrinkles or soft spots.

Prep: Rinse and chop, you can keep the skin on or peel it. For most aubergine dishes people don't use the skin. However, it is edible, so if you want to give it a try, you can eat it.

Cook: To help soften aubergine before cooking it, chop it and generously sea salt it in a colander and let stand for 5–10 minutes. Rinse off the sea salt before cooking. **On the stove:** Chop the aubergine into cubes, add to a warm skillet with coconut oil and fresh parsley, and cook for about 5 minutes. **In the oven:** Preheat the oven to 200°C/400°F/gas 6. Brush the aubergine slices with coconut oil and arrange on a baking sheet in a single layer. Cook for about 15 minutes, turning halfway through. **On the grill:** Brush the aubergine slices with coconut oil and place under a medium heat for about 8 minutes, turning once.

Avocado

Looks like: a thick, deep green or black skin, should feel a little tender when you squeeze it.

Prep: Rinse and slice lengthwise around the pit, then put down the knife and hold the avocado in your hands to twist the two halves apart. Remove the pit by scooping it out with a spoon, or leave it in if you are only eating half the avocado, as it will help to prevent the remaining flesh browning.

Raw: You can easily spread it on sandwiches or veggie burgers by mashing it before you spread, or slice it into salads.

Beetroot (Beet)

Looks like: a little dirty, rough-skinned on the outside, with a dark ruby or bright orange inner skin.

Prep: Wash and peel off outer skin.

Raw: You can eat beetroot raw (especially in salad); simply use a veggie peeler to remove the tough outer skin and then shred the inner flesh into small pieces.

Cook: If you enjoy cooked beetroots, just give them a quick rinse, add a little coconut oil and sea salt to the outside, wrap in tin foil and bake in the oven (skins on), for 45 minutes–1 hour at 200°C/400°F/gas 6. Once done, the skin will easily fall off and you have a delicious beetroot that you can cut to your preferred size or shape. Try slicing them on top of a salad.

Bok choy

Looks like: a bunch of white stems and leafy green tops – watch out for any wilting or yellowing leaves.

Prep: Chop off the base of the plant to make it easier to rinse and be sure to rub the stalks to remove any dirt or grit.

Raw: You can slice stalks and leaves and add to an Asian-inspired salad with fresh mint leaves and lime juice.

Cook: This hearty green goes great in stir-fries or as its own side dish – simply chop it and add to any stovetop dish. **On the stove:** Bring a pan of water to a boil and add the bok choy for about 2 minutes. Remove, then toss in a little sesame oil, brown rice vinegar and soy sauce.

Broccoli

Looks like: little green trees, go for a high floret-to-stem ratio with no yellowing, should feel firm to the touch.

Prep: Rinse and chop off the florets. You can cut the stalks in half lengthwise and then into half-moons.

Raw: Chopped florets go great in salads or with hummus and other veggie dips.

Cook: Goes great in stir-fries and soups. **Steam:** Place stems in a steamer basket above 2in/5cm of water in a large pan on a high heat. Cover and steam for 2–3 minutes. Add the florets, cover and leave to steam for another 5 minutes. Toss with fresh lemon juice, olive oil and sea salt. **In the oven:** Preheat the oven to 200°C/400°F/gas 6. Spread the florets on a baking sheet in a single layer and coat with coconut oil and sea salt. Cook for about 10 minutes, turning once halfway through.

Brussels sprouts

Looks like: little cabbage heads, look for freshness by avoiding yellow or tattered leaves.

Prep: Rinse, remove any tough outer leaves and trim the stem.

Cook: Steam: Place the sprouts in a steamer basket over 2in/5cm of water in a large pan on a high heat. Cover and steam for 5–7 minutes. **In the oven:** Preheat the oven to 200°C/400°F/gas 6. Cut the sprouts in half, spread on a baking sheet in a single layer, and coat with coconut oil and sea salt. Roast for about 20 minutes, turning once halfway through.

Butternut squash

Looks like: a longer squash with a light orange skin.

Prep: Rinse and cut lengthwise, scoop out the seeds and stringy bits with a spoon.

Cook: Steam: Preheat the oven to 180°C/350°F/gas 4. Place the squash, cut side down, in a baking dish.

Add 4fl oz/125ml/½ cup of water and then cover tightly with foil. Bake for 1 hour. Remove from the oven and let cool. Scoop out the squash and mash the flesh with coconut oil and sea salt. **In the oven:** Slice the butternut squash into half-moon slices, or dice it. Toss with coconut oil, honey and cinnamon and roast at 200°C/400°F/gas 6 for about 40 minutes.

Quick tip: You can find butternut squash already sliced in many supermarkets, during the autumn, or canned and mashed.

Cabbage

Looks like: compact, round head of sturdy leaves – can be green or red, the outer leaves should not be discoloured or shrivelled.

Prep: Remove the outer leaves and rinse. Cut the cabbage in half, slicing through the stem, and remove the core.

Raw: You can thinly slice it or shred it with a knife or use a food processor. It's a great base for a healthier coleslaw dressed with mustard and fresh orange juice rather than mayo.

Cook: Goes great in stir-fries, soups and stews. **Steam/ Boil:** Bring about 1in/2.5cm of water to the boil in a large pan, and add the cabbage wedges and salt. Simmer, covered, for 8–10 minutes. Sprinkle the boiled cabbage with sea salt, pepper and extra virgin olive oil to serve.

Cauliflower

Looks like: a head of little white trees, go for a high floret-to-stem ratio with no yellowing, they should feel firm to the touch.

Prep: Rinse and chop off the florets. Sometimes it's easiest to start by chopping the head in half, then into quarters.

Raw: Chopped florets go great with hummus and other veggie dips.

Cook: Goes great in stir-fries and soups. **Steam:** Place stems in a steamer basket above 2in/5cm of water in a large pan over a high heat. Cover and steam for 2–3 minutes. Add the florets, then cover and steam for another 5 minutes. Toss with fresh lemon juice, olive oil and sea salt. **In the oven:** Preheat the oven to 200°C/400°F/gas 6. Spread the florets on a baking sheet in a single layer and coat with coconut oil and sea salt. Cook for about 15 minutes, turning once halfway through.

Carrot

Looks like: Firm, orange spear, preferably with greens at the end.

Prep: Cut off the greens, peel and rinse thoroughly.

Raw: Chop into bite-size chunks for hummus and veggie dips. Carrot can be puréed into a carrot-ginger dressing for salads too.

Cook: Carrots are quite versatile in the kitchen, and they make a great base for almost any soup, stew or sauce. **In the oven:** Preheat the oven to 200°C/400°F/ gas 6. Cut the carrots in half lengthwise and slice into half-moon pieces. Spread on a baking sheet in a single layer and coat with coconut oil. Roast for about 15 minutes. **On the stove:** Chop the carrots into half-moon pieces and sauté in a pan with a little bit of coconut oil over a medium heat for about 5 minutes. Season with sea salt and fresh parsley. **Steam:** Chop the carrots into smaller pieces and place in a large pot in a steamer basket set above 1in/2.5cm of water. Put on a high heat and cover and steam for 5 minutes.

Celeriac (Celery root)

Looks like: an unusual-looking, off-white, round root veggie.

Prep: Rinse and remove the base and top with a knife. To peel it, cut down the sides, close to the skin.

Raw: You can thinly slice it into matchsticks or grate it coarsely and toss it into a salad.

Cook: In the oven: Make your own celeriac chips. Simply slice the whole thing in half and then quarters and slice each quarter as thinly as you can. Toss the pieces in coconut oil, sprinkle with sea salt, spread onto a baking sheet in one layer (may require 2 sheets). Roast the rounds at 180°C/350°F/gas 4 until they are golden brown, about 15–20 minutes.

On the stove: Make a hearty soup by cubing celeriac and mixing with potatoes, leeks and veggie broth. Simmer ingredients on the stove for 30 minutes and then blend with a hand blender. Top it with a drizzle of extra virgin olive oil and thinly sliced scallions.

Celery

Looks like: long green stems, which should be firm, topped with fresh leaves.

Prep: Rinse and chop off the stem.

Raw: Chop into bite-size chunks for hummus and veggie dips. Goes great thinly sliced and added to any kind of chopped salad.

Cook: Slice and use in veggie stir-fries, broths or stews. **On the stove:** You can braise celery by simply adding slices to veggie broth in a saucepan and simmering on low for 10–15 minutes.

Quick tip: Celery leaves are edible and delicious – use them in soups and stews.

Chard

Looks like: long stems with green tops, stem colours can be white, red or yellow.

Prep: Chop off the base of the plant and separate the stems for washing. You can fill a large bowl with cool water and put a bunch of chard in the bowl – all the grit will sink to the bottom.

Raw: Roll the leaves into a cigar shape and thinly slice. Toss into a salad with lemon and olive oil.

Cook: Chard is a mild-tasting green and goes well in stir-fries and pasta dishes. **On the stove:** Slice stems and leaves and add the stems to the pan first with a drop of coconut oil or water. Cook for 3–5 minutes and then add the leaves and cook for another 5 minutes. Drizzle with olive oil, lemon juice and sea salt.

Corn

Looks like: bright green outer husks, each ear should feel firm to touch. On the inside corn can be white, yellow, blue, red or a variety of colours.

Prep: Pull back the husks and remove, rinse the ears.

Raw: Remove kernels from the cobs and add to a salad or eat right off the cob.

Cook: Corn is great at a barbecue, whether it's on the grill or in a salad. **Grill:** Pull back the husks without removing them and pull out the silks. Soak the ears in water for 20 minutes. Place corn in husks over a high heat and grill, turning occasionally, for about 5 minutes. **Steam:** Husk the corn, then cut the ears in half. Place the corn in 2in/5cm of water in a large pot on a high heat. Cover and steam for 4–5 minutes.

Courgette (Zucchini) and summer squash

Looks like: a long green tube with a stem at the top; summer squash is yellow.

Prep: Wash and remove the stem.

Raw: Use a spiralizer to make raw zucchini noodles or shred and toss into salads. (A spiralizer is a tool that is used to make long ribbons from vegetables, you can pick one up at a cooking store. If you can't get one, slice the courgette in a food processor, or with a mandolin, or use a sharp knife to make thin strips.)

Cook: This classic Italian veggie goes great in pasta dishes. **In the oven:** Slice into rounds and spread on a baking sheet in a single layer. Drizzle coconut oil and ground almond flour on top and bake for 20 minutes. **On the grill:** Marinate in lemon juice, coconut oil and garlic for at least 20 minutes, then grill at a medium heat for a few minutes on each side.

Cucumber

Looks like: a long green tube, some varieties are shorter (like Kirby) and others are longer (English) – make sure it's firm to the touch.

Prep: Rinse and dry. You can peel cucumbers, but if you are buying organic eat the skin as it is good for you.

Raw: Slice, dice, chop in any way and add to salads or just enjoy cucumber slices with a little lime and paprika sprinkled over.

Dandelion

Looks like: rocket (arugula) but with longer, pointier leaves.

Prep: Wash dandelion leaves by placing them in a large bowl with cool water and swish the leaves around to remove the dirt. You can chop off the roots and stalks.

Raw: You can add dandelion to salads, but be warned it has a bitter flavour. You're better off cooking dandelion, if you're new to it. It does go well in a fresh pesto with basil, lemon, olive oil and pumpkin seeds.

Cook: On the stove: Add a little coconut oil or veggie broth to a pan and sauté greens with chopped garlic for about 5 minutes.

Fennel

Looks like: small, white bulbs with green stalks and feathery fronds, smells like liquorice.

Prep: Chop off the stalks and fronds at the point where they meet the bulb. Cut the bulb in half and remove the core.

Raw: Slice thinly and add to salads.

Cook: **On the stove:** Add sliced fennel pieces to a large pan with coconut oil or veggie broth, along with some dried rosemary and lemon juice. Let the mixture simmer for about 15 minutes, adding more broth as you need it. **In the oven:** Preheat the oven to 200°C/400°F/gas 6. Spread the fennel slices on a baking sheet in a single layer. Coat with coconut oil and cook for about 20 minutes.

Green beans

Looks like: thin, firm green tubes with a stem.

Prep: Rinse and snap off the stem with your hand.

Cook: **Steam:** Put beans in a steamer basket over about 1in/2.5cm of water in a large pan on a high heat. Cover and steam for 5 minutes. **On the stove:** Heat a little bit of coconut oil or vegetable broth in a large skillet. Add the beans and cook, stirring occasionally, for about 3 minutes. Add a squeeze of lemon and a handful of toasted almonds or pecans and serve warm.

Kale

Looks like: long, dark green, leafy bunches, some varieties have purple or red hues.

Prep: Rinse thoroughly under running water. You can easily separate the kale from its stem by holding it stem-side up and pulling off the leaves with your hands.

Then you can ribbon chop the kale by rolling it into a cigar shape and thinly slicing it.

Raw: Goes great in salads. The trick is to massage the kale first with your hands and a little extra virgin olive oil. This helps break down the veggie, making it a little sweeter.

Cook: Kale is a great addition to stir-fries, soups and sauces. **Steam:** To reduce its bitterness, simply add kale to a pan of boiling water for a minute or two and drain. Top with your favourite Reboot-friendly dressing. **On the stove**: Add a bunch of kale to a pan with veggie broth or water and simmer for about 15 minutes. Dress with olive oil, lemon and sea salt.

Leek

Looks like: long, wide green stalks that are not bruised; should not be wrinkly.

Prep: Trim off the top thick green leaves, leaving the pale green and white parts. Remove any damaged outer layers. Split in half lengthwise. Rinse under cold running water.

Cook: Leeks are a great substitute for onion in any dish. **On the stove**: Add chopped leeks to a large pan with veggie broth, garlic and rosemary and simmer for about 10 minutes. **On the grill:** Brush leeks with coconut oil and place under a medium heat until lightly browned, about 5 minutes.

Lettuce

Looks like: big leafy greens, come in many varieties from romaine to bibb to green or red leaf.

Prep: Rinse thoroughly under running water and dry off either with a paper towel or in a salad spinner.

Raw: Romaine leaves are sturdy enough for a lettuce wrap to be filled with hummus or any veggie dip. Chop lettuce leaves to make a great salad with a Reboot-friendly dressing.

Mushrooms

Looks like: white, brown or earth-coloured caps or buttons (with or without stems).

Prep: Use a damp paper towel or cloth to remove dirt from mushrooms, trim stems when needed.

Cook: Mushrooms go great in veggie stir-fries as they add a little extra moisture to the mix. **On the stove:** Heat a little bit of coconut oil in pan over a medium heat, add sliced mushrooms and a pinch of sea salt. Cook for 8–10 minutes, stirring occasionally.

Onion

Looks like: white, yellow or red bulbs with flaky skin, be sure they don't have soft spots.

Prep: Trim off the stem end first. Remove the dry,

papery skin with your hands; it can help to make a shallow cut down the side of the onion into the first layer and then peel. Leave the root end intact, cut the onion lengthwise and begin cutting the onion into quarters and then slice, eventually removing the root.

Raw: Red onion can make for a pretty topping on a salad, or a little diced onion on a veggie burger always spices things up.

Cook: Add chopped onions to a pan as the base of almost any meal. **On the stove:** Add a little coconut oil or veggie broth to a pan on a medium heat. Add the onions and sauté for 5 minutes.

Parsnip

Looks like: a white carrot.

Prep: Trim the root and leaf and scrub well.

Raw: Chop up like a carrot, peel and serve with hummus or a veggie dip.

Cook: In the oven: Preheat the oven to 200°C/400°F/ gas 6. Cut the parsnips in half lengthwise and slice into half-moon pieces. Spread on a baking sheet in a single layer and coat with coconut oil and sea salt. Roast for about 15 minutes. **On the stove:** Add chopped parsnips to a pan with a little bit of coconut oil over a medium heat and sauté for about 5 minutes. Season with sea salt and fresh parsley. **Steam:** Chop parsnips into smaller pieces and place in a steamer basket set above 1in/2.5cm of water in a large pot on high heat. Cover and steam for 5 minutes.

Pumpkin

Looks like: a big orange ball with a stem. For cooking purposes, choose a smaller variety like sugar pumpkin.

Prep: Rinse and slice in half starting from the stem and moving down. Scoop out the seeds and stringy bits. Rinse off the seeds and bake for homemade pumpkin seeds.

Cook: In the oven: Preheat oven to 180°C/350°F/gas 4. Place the pumpkin halves on a baking sheet or in a baking tin, add ½in/1.5cm of water and bake uncovered for 1 hour. Remove from the oven and allow to cool. When cool, scoop out the insides to mash or use in any recipe that calls for pumpkin purée.

Quick tip: You can buy canned pumpkin, just be sure it doesn't have added sugars or preservatives.

Radish

Looks like: small red or white bulbs.

Prep: Rinse and remove the roots and leaves.

Raw: You can serve them whole, sliced or diced with hummus or other veggie dips. You can grate them over a salad.

Cook: You can pickle them! For a quick recipe: quarter 6 radishes and toss with sea salt in a bowl and let stand for 30 minutes. Add 3 tablespoons of rice vinegar, 2 tablespoons honey and a 1-in/2.5-cm piece of ginger to a saucepan over medium heat, stirring until the honey is dissolved. Stir in radishes. Transfer to a small bowl and leave to marinate for at least 2 hours.

Rocket (Arugula)

Looks like: a small lettuce with curly leaves; look for crisp colourful leaves, not wilted or yellow.

Prep: This green can be quite sandy, so give it a good rinse before using. You can fill a large bowl with cool water and swish the rocket around in the bowl and all the grit will sink to the bottom.

Raw: Rocket is great in salads or as a substitute for lettuce in a wrap. It will add a peppery and sometimes spicy flavour.

Cook: You can also toss the leaves into a warm salad or pasta dish for an extra dash of green colour and nutrition. It cooks very quickly, so add in the last few minutes of cooking.

Spaghetti squash

Looks like: large, yellow tube with a stem, usually about 12in/30cm long.

Prep: Give it a rinse and pierce it with a fork in several spots to prepare it for baking.

Cook: This squash works as a great alternative to pasta because the cooked squash easily shreds into thin spaghetti-like strands. **In the oven:** Place the whole squash in a baking tin and bake at 190°C/375°F/gas 5 for 1 hour. Let it cool for about 20 minutes, then cut it in half lengthwise. Just like other squash, scoop out the seeds and stringy bits in the centre. Use a fork to gently scrape around the edges of the squash and work toward the middle to create strands. Serve it with olive oil and sea salt or top it with your favourite tomato sauce.

Spinach

Looks like: small, dark green leaves.

Prep: Rinse thoroughly under running water or fill a big bowl with cool water and swish spinach leaves around – any dirt will fall to the bottom.

Raw: Spinach salad is a classic!

Cook: Add spinach to any dish for a little extra colour, but know that spinach cooks down a lot. If you're serving it as a side dish use twice or three times the amount you think you'll need. **On the stove:** Add leaves to a pan with a drop of coconut oil or water. Cook for about 3 minutes. Drizzle with olive oil and sea salt.

Quick tip: Buy ready washed spinach in a bag and save time rinsing.

Spring greens (Collard greens)

Looks like: short thick stalks and large, wide green leaves – watch out for yellowing leaves.

Prep: Wash these greens by plunging them into a cool bowl of water or gently rubbing them under running water.

Raw: Spring greens work great as a substitute for bread. You can remove the stem and use the leaf to make a delicious veggie wrap. You can also lightly steam the leaves for a few minutes to soften them and take away the mild grassy flavour.

Cook: You can quickly chop the greens by stacking 5 leaves on top of each other and rolling them into a cigar. Then slice them into small strips. **On the stove:** Sauté the thinly sliced strips with vegetable broth, chopped garlic and onion for about 10 minutes over a medium heat. Serve hot as a side dish.

Spring onions (Scallions)

Looks like: a long green stem with a small white bulb at the end.

Prep: Be sure to rinse stems thoroughly and rinse inside the green part of the scallion.

Raw: Chop into small slices and scatter over soups and salads.

Cook: Add the green part of scallions to garnish a

soup, such as miso, or add to stir-fry dishes for extra flavour.

Sprouts

Looks like: small green leaves with long stems.

Prep: You can find anything from broccoli to alfalfa in sprout form. Rinse them thoroughly and enjoy on top of salads or in wraps.

Sugar snap peas

Looks like: fresh green pods with small peas inside and stems.

Prep: Rinse and snap off the stems with your hands.

Raw: Goes great with hummus and other veggie dips.

Cook: Sugar snap peas are best in stir-fries. **On the stove:** Heat veggie broth in a pan over a medium heat and cook for about 3 minutes. They will turn bright green.

Sweet (bell) pepper (Capsicum)

Looks like: bright green, orange, red or yellow bell-shape. Look for firm peppers with shiny skin.

Prep: Rinse and slice. You can start by holding the pepper, stem-up, and cut into quarters, removing the white pith and seeds from the centre.

Raw: You can enjoy peppers in a salad, simply slice and dice as you like.

Cook: Peppers go great in a veggie chilli or a pasta dish. **On the grill:** Put peppers on the grill until they are blackened, then peel off the charred outer skin and enjoy the sweet roasted peppers on their own or with some fresh garlic and olive oil.

Sweet potato

Looks like: an orange potato, should be very firm to the touch.

Prep: Scrub off any dirt. You can peel them, but then you will miss out on the nutrients and fibre.

Cook: In the oven: Make your own sweet potato fries! Preheat oven to 230°C/450°F/gas 8. Slice the potatoes into wedges, put them in a big bowl and coat with coconut oil, sea salt and chilli powder, then spread them on a baking sheet in one layer. Bake for 20–25 minutes, occasionally turning them. **Steam:** Cut into 1-in/2.5-cm pieces and place in a steamer basket set over 2in/5cm of water in a pan on a high heat. Cover and steam for about 20 minutes. For mashed sweet potatoes, simply add almond milk and olive oil to the mixture.

Quick tip: You can find canned sweet potato, just be sure it doesn't have added sugars or preservatives.

Tomato

Looks like: a big red bulb, also comes in green, yellow, or stripey; cherry tomatoes are the smaller, bite-size version.

Prep: Wash and chop off the top with the stem, then cut into slices. For a finer chop, keep going and slice and dice until you have cubes.

Raw: Tomatoes go great in salads, on top of a veggie burger, or diced in a fresh salsa.

Cook: You can use fresh tomatoes to make a pasta sauce or in veggie soup, like minestrone. **In the oven:** Try slow-roasting tomatoes to get their full sweetness. Preheat the oven to 160°C/325°F/gas 3. Spread the tomato slices on a baking sheet in a single layer and drizzle over some coconut oil and sprinkle with sea salt. Cook for 2 hours – perfect for a day when you are at home doing chores.

Turnip

Looks like: very firm, red and white skins in a bulb shape, can have greens attached at the top.

Prep: Rinse and chop off the root end and the greens. You can peel and then cut into slices.

Cook: On the stove: Cut the turnip into matchstick slices. Add a little coconut oil to a pan over a medium heat, add the slices and cook for about 10 minutes, stirring often. **In the oven:** Preheat the oven to 240°C/475°F/gas 9 and spread the turnip slices on a baking sheet in a single layer. Coat with coconut oil, sprinkle with sea salt and cook for about 15 minutes.

Basic cooking techniques explained

- **Baking:** Place food in the oven, either on a baking sheet or in a covered or uncovered glass baking dish or other oven-safe cookware, e.g. cast iron.

- **Barbecuing:** With this technique, food is placed on a rack over heat applied from below. The process imparts a distinctive charred flavour. Avoid over-charring animal proteins, as this can create carcinogens.

- **Grilling (Broiling):** This is done with heat applied from above. It is a great alternative to frying because it requires very little fat and gives food a crisp outside.

- **Roasting:** Similar to baking, but at higher temperatures. When roasting vegetables, line a baking sheet or roasting pan with baking parchment to make the subsequent cleaning easier.

- **Sautéing:** using a very hot pan on the stove top with a small amount of fat (we like coconut oil) to quickly cook food while browning the surface.

- **Steaming:** Use a steamer or place a steaming basket over simmering liquid on the hob. It's best to steam vegetables lightly so that they maintain their colour and crispness.

- **Stir-frying:** Heat a small amount of oil in a non-stick pan or wok. When hot, add small pieces of food (all roughly the same size) and stir rapidly with a wooden spoon or spatula. The aim is to cook food lightly and maintain its natural colour and texture.

HOW TO PREPARE LEAFY GREENS

Leafy greens have many virtues. They are nutritional power-houses packed with vitamins and antioxidants. They cook up relatively quickly and are pretty tasty too. Unfortunately, they are still one of the most missing ingredients in many people's diets. You may have seen them in a store in all their fresh, crispy glory, but you may feel intimidated when it comes to knowing how to prepare them. Here's an easy guide to get you started.

In a juice: Just rinse, soak in cold water to remove excess dirt and grit, then push through your juicer's feeder tube and enjoy.

In a smoothie: Add fresh chopped greens to your favourite smoothie recipe for a nutrient boost. Try banana, almond milk, frozen strawberries and a handful of spinach or kale for a quick breakfast or afternoon snack.

In a salad: For thin leafy greens like spinach, lightly toss them with your favourite dressing and top with nuts or seeds. I enjoy heartier greens like kale best when they are chopped in little pieces, stems removed, and massaged with a little olive oil or avocado for a silkier texture and a sweeter flavour.

In soups and stews: Stir leafy greens into your favourite soup or stew to add a little green to the mix. Try in a lentil soup or even in a heartier potato and leek version.

In a stir-fry: Toss chopped greens such as bok choy, kale or cabbage into a stir-fry and cook for an additional 5 minutes before serving.

Steam/boil: You can retain more of your greens' brilliant colour and more nutrients with a quick dunk in a large skillet-type pan. Here's how: Take about 16fl oz/500ml/2 cups of water for one bunch of greens. Bring the water to a boil first and add a little sea salt. Then add the washed, chopped greens and cook on a medium heat, covered, for 3–10 minutes, depending on the type of green you are cooking – as a general rule, the more bitter the flavour, the longer you should cook them. When you drain the greens, keep the water as a broth or just drink it.

Sauté: Greens are great on the stove and cook up quick. Try chopped spinach, kale, chard, spring greens (collard) or rocket (arugula) in a pan with a little coconut oil, garlic, lemon juice and sea salt. They cook up in 3–5 minutes for a great side dish. Raisins and pine nuts are great on top of greens and help complement the bitter flavour.

Bake/chips: Kale chips are an amazing substitute for potato chips. Simply rinse the kale, tear into smaller pieces and add coconut oil, sea salt and paprika. Spread the kale on a baking sheet in a single layer and cook for 15 minutes at 180°C/350F/gas 4.

What to do with chopped stems: While you may be tempted to throw away your green stems, consider adding them to an omelette or stir-fry, or simply sauté them in a pan with some coconut oil for a few minutes and then add them to your favourite dish.

Feeding the family while Rebooting

It's a bit ironic that many Rebooters are motivated to get healthy by their kids, but it is their kids that get in the way of a successful Reboot. It's not facing temptation when you sit down at the dinner table and you're the only one with the glass of liquid sunshine that's the problem, it's the extra work of preparing both dinner for them and juices for you. Here are some of the most helpful tips I've heard along the way from Rebooters all over the world:

1 If you're eating on your Reboot, let your family eat what you eat. Make enough of what you eat to feed the whole family but maybe add in a lean protein or whole grain to their dish. The recipes are selected carefully so that everyone can enjoy them, and you won't even miss the protein or the whole grains.

2 If you're just juicing, try incorporating the same fruits and veggies that you're drinking into dinner – you can juice sweet potatoes while the rest of the family has roast sweet potatoes.

3 Or, juice until dinner then eat the cooked veggies, while your family has additional grains and proteins.

4 When it's time to sit down at the dinner table, drink another juice while your family eats, and concentrate on drinking it slowly. You could even do the chewing motion with your teeth to slow down the pace.

5 Check out our pulp recipes for delicious ways you can use that leftover pulp. Your family will be getting so many added nutrients and half the time they won't even notice. Carrots and beetroots are excellent for Veggie Burgers (see p. 229)!

6 Have a juice on hand to enjoy while you are cooking to keep you full and your mind off all the smells that are coming out of your kitchen.

7 If being surrounded by your family's food is just too hard for you, ask your partner or your children to take over in the kitchen while you Reboot. Or find healthy take-away options for them and drink your juice alone while the family eats. It's OK if that's the only way you can say no to food!

Everyone is different, just listen to yourself and find the way that helps you stay committed.

Rebooting for thyroid conditions

A question often asked on our Ask the Nutritionist forum is 'what fruits and vegetables should I avoid if I have a thyroid condition?' This is because it has been shown that some vegetables can interfere with the way thyroid hormones are manufactured by the thyroid gland.

Your thyroid is a butterfly-shaped gland that sits near your vocal cords and produces thyroid hormones that control your metabolism. Symptoms of an under-active thyroid gland can be low body temperature, constipation, weight gain, hair loss, dry flaky skin and nails, fluid retention, slow reflexes, fatigue and slow thoughts and cognition. Thyroid problems can develop for a number of reasons, but the most common causes are nutrient deficiencies such as iodine and selenium deficiency, auto-immune disease, genetics, stress and environmental factors. The most common type of thyroid problem is hypothyroidism (under-active gland).

The concern for anyone with a thyroid issue who is Rebooting is that eating raw cruciferous vegetables can further suppress your thyroid hormone function and may also interfere with your body's ability to lose weight. So, if you have a thyroid issue pay close attention to your veggies. Avoid consuming LARGE amounts of RAW cruciferous vegetables including broccoli, cauliflower, Brussels sprouts, bok choy, broccolini, Chinese cabbage, kale, kohlrabi, radish, mustard greens, spring (collard) greens, choy sum, horseradish and turnips.

This means you'll need to make some modifications to your juice – take my Mean Green, for example. Rather than including kale, substitute spinach or romaine instead and add more cucumber, courgettes (zucchini) or celery for that extra green. Cruciferous vegetables are certainly healthy and have been shown to support the liver in its natural detoxification processes, so if you are doing a juicing plus eating Reboot, have these vegetables cooked instead of raw. And eat them cooked when you've finished your Reboot!

It is important to note that if you have a normal thyroid function and consume adequate amounts of iodine, these vegetables will have no effect on your thyroid, meaning that for anyone with a healthy thyroid, juicing lots of kale won't cause a thyroid problem. These modifications are only necessary for those with an existing condition.

If you have a thyroid condition, follow these healthy tips for a plant-based diet anytime, whether you are Rebooting or not:

1 **All fruits and vegetables** contain powerful phytonutrients that support a healthy immune system. Due to the inflammation seen in an auto-immune disease, it is important to reduce the inflammation with antioxidants by eating a rainbow to provide valuable phytonutrients.

2 Eating **selenium**-rich foods such as Brazil nuts, shellfish, eggs, sunflower seeds and garlic will help to support a healthy metabolism. Selenium content varies in foods depending on the soil content – some geographical regions are very low. Selenium deficiency can be determined with a red blood cell selenium blood test, otherwise by hair and nail analysis.

3 Healthy thyroid function also requires adequate levels of **iodine,** a trace mineral, which is required by the body for the synthesis of thyroid hormones. Eat iodine-rich foods such as seaweed, marine fish, pineapple, iodized sea salt (avoid the free-flowing agent), spinach and lettuce.

4 **Stress** can be a big factor that has a negative impact on your thyroid hormones and can fire up auto-immune activity. Commit yourself to stress-management techniques such as meditation, yoga, warm baths, exercise, reading and other relaxing activities.

5 **Excess fluoride and bromide** exposure can interfere with the health of the thyroid. Fluoride and bromide can be taken into the thyroid gland in place of iodine.

6 **Avoid gluten if you are intolerant.** There are a number of studies that indicate auto-immune diseases, particularly Hashimoto's disease, can be related to a gluten intolerance or coeliac disease. You can find more information on gluten intolerance and coeliac disease on www.rebootwithjoe.com.

7 **Avoid** sugar, caffeine, refined processed foods, preservatives, additives and synthetic colours as much as possible.

8 **Coconut oil** has shown particular promise in some studies to help stimulate a sluggish thyroid.

So go ahead and feel empowered with a sluggish thyroid gland. With a few modifications to your Reboot, you can succeed in excellent energy, health and weight-loss goals.

Rebooting for diabetes

Diabetes is a disease where blood sugar levels are higher than normal or above a healthy range. The body produces the hormone insulin to move glucose/sugar into our cells. In diabetes sufferers, the body either doesn't produce enough insulin or can't use the insulin it makes well enough and so sugars build up in the blood.

The obesity epidemic, diabetes, insulin resistance and pre-diabetes all go hand in hand. According to Diabetes UK, in 2012 around 3 million people, 4.6 per cent of the population, in the UK were found to have diabetes.[6] The Australian Government's Institute of Health and Welfare estimated that in 2012, there were 999,000 Australians with a diagnosis of diabetes and over half the adult population were found to be overweight, putting them at risk of diabetes.[7]

The detrimental effects of diabetes are mind-blowing.

It is a major cause of heart disease, stroke and the leading cause of kidney failure, lower limb amputations (non-trauma related), new cases of blindness and the seventh leading cause of death. People with diabetes have twice the risk for depression and depression itself can increase the risk of type 2 diabetes by 60 per cent. Diabetes can lead to complications with pregnancy, increased risk of infections or more difficult and complicated recovery from illness, dental diseases, and also raised blood pressure and cholesterol levels. High levels of insulin in the blood or insulin resistance are being linked to increased risk for certain cancers and higher probability of cancer recurrence in survivors.

The encouraging news is that up to 93 per cent of diabetes cases may be preventable with a healthy lifestyle. And many Rebooters with diabetes have successfully participated in both juice-only and juice-plus-food, jumpstarting into a healthy lifestyle and even decreasing and sometimes eliminating the need for medications.

But if you have diabetes it's important to customise your Reboot plan and take certain factors into consideration, and always to consult with your doctor before starting a Reboot. For anyone with type 1 diabetes or those taking insulin or other diabetes medications, it is especially important to discuss how to adjust your medication appropriately during your Reboot. (For more information see our advice on talking to your doctor: For Your Doctor, p. 244.)

If you have diabetes, we recommend modifying your Reboot:

- Consider the 10-Day Reboot plan or the first 5 days of the 15-Day Classic Reboot which includes eating + juicing. The extra fibre from whole vegetables and fruits will help keep blood sugar steady.

- Include blended vegetables/fruits. Fibre from complex carbohydrates in the form of whole foods is KEY, it will help keep sugar levels steady and making your smoothie or blend with mostly vegetables will also lower the total carbohydrate amount while keeping the nutrient levels high.

- Pay extra attention to hydration and drink plenty of water. When you're dehydrated your blood is more concentrated and sugar levels can be higher.

- Stay active – exercise has its own way of helping to keep blood sugar levels in check. While strength training is important, regular cardiovascular exercise has been shown to have the greatest positive impact on diabetic patients. Learn more about the Reboot Movement Method and discover ideas for healthy activities during your Reboot at www.RebootwithJoe.com/fitness.

- Create your juices with more veggies compared to fruits. Be sure to follow our tried and true 80/20 rule of 80 per cent veggies and 20 per cent fruits.

- Look for juices that have diabetes listed in the 'Good For' next to the recipes in this book, these are lower in sugar and carbohydrates.

And here our top five tips for managing diabetes, whether on a Reboot or not:

1 Eat small, frequent meals throughout the day. Eating this way can help keep blood sugar levels stable and prevent overeating, which in turn promotes weight management. (Maintaining or working towards a healthy weight is so crucial for anyone with type 2 diabetes.)

2 Pair protein with carbohydrate-rich foods, including fruits and starchy veggies. Protein- and fibre-rich foods are digested more slowly than carbohydrate-rich foods, making this combination key for keeping blood sugar levels stable and within a healthy range. Adding protein to carbs helps to slow the absorption of sugar from the carbohydrate-rich foods. For example, almond butter on apple slices or a handful of almonds with an orange.

3 Eat a fruit or veggie with every meal and snack. Increasing your intake of fruits and vegetables helps to provide a healthy balance of nutrients like fibre, vitamins, minerals and a wealth of phytonutrients. Eating whole fruits and vegetables helps control blood sugar, for example it takes three whole oranges to raise your blood sugar to the same level as just 6oz/180ml of commercial, pasteurised orange juice. For fresh juices out of your juicer we suggest more veggie-based juices.

4 Drink plenty of water; being dehydrated raises blood sugar levels by making your blood more

concentrated. Hydration helps boost energy levels, reduce sugary cravings and supports metabolism.

5 Include cinnamon in your diet. Research suggests that cinnamon can help keep blood sugar levels in check. Try sprinkling some into your favourite meals, including smoothies, fresh juice and even chilli!

After your Reboot

When you have big health goals, you might need a drastic change in your diet to help you get there, and a Reboot is an excellent way to reset your system. It's what ultimately saved my life and set me up to remain on this path that has kept me 70 pounds lighter than when I started and, most importantly, medication free.

Sometimes I have to remind myself that I only drank fruit and vegetable juice for 60 days followed by 90 days of only eating and juicing fruits and vegetables. It still sounds pretty extreme, but my goals were extreme, and in the end I was able to achieve extreme results. At the end of that journey, I was able to look at myself in the mirror and recognise the person staring back at me – the energetic, athletic, healthy mate I once was – and I looked at my medicine cabinet and said, 'Sayonara!'

While the benefits of a Reboot are countless, a Reboot is not a sustainable diet to maintain for the rest of your life. Our bodies need the right balance of protein, healthy fats, insoluble fibre and a variety of plant-based foods to function properly over the long term. The beauty of a Reboot is that once it's done, you can still incorporate juices and heaps of fruits and vegetables throughout your daily life to maintain all the great benefits of a Reboot – clear skin, energy, weight loss and health improvements – and continue to be in the driver's seat on the road to optimal health. But how to incorporate healthy proteins and fats and an occasional treat in to your diet without backsliding into your old diet is where things can get a little tricky.

If you step into the diet and health section at a bookstore today there are hundreds of different diets that promise you weight loss, health and a fabulous physique. It's confusing to know which one to follow once you come off your Reboot. Well, let me tell you this. You don't need to follow one specific plan. You don't need to put a stamp on your eating habits by identifying yourself as raw, vegan, vegetarian, paleo, gluten-free, dairy-free, macrobiotic, pescetarian . . . I could go on and on.

However, if this helps you to stick to a diet that works right for you then by all means, go for it. I don't have a problem with any of these diets, nor do I endorse one over the other. It's up to you to determine what diet works for you. For me, a diet that is high in fruit and vegetables along with fish and meat a few times a week, and chocolate ice cream once every seven to ten days, works best. I stay away from gluten as I notice

I tend to gain weight if I eat bread, and I have at least one juice pretty much daily.

When you come off your Reboot, start adding in foods that you think are good for your lifestyle to find out what works for you. You may find that a diet filled with lots of plants and the occasional meats, a grass-fed yoghurt here or there is best for you. Or you may find it is easier for you to sustain your health gains by eating vegan. And what's best for you is the best diet out there. In the resource section, I've included a list of recipe books that have been inspirational and informative for Rebooters trying to determine their diet for life.

The recipes in this book are meant for Rebooting but are also excellent as part of an after-the-Reboot diet. They are a great way to continue consuming heaps of fruits and vegetables, and if you want to add something more, you can always incorporate wild fish, free-range organic chicken, grass-fed beef or anything else you enjoy, such as quinoa or brown rice. There are also tons of plant-based recipes at www.rebootwithjoe.com.

DIETS DEFINED

Dairy-free: People following a dairy-free diet avoid anything with cow's, sheep's or goat's milk products, including milk, cheese and yoghurt. Dairy is a common allergen. Many other diets are also daiary-free.

Gluten-free: A gluten-free diet (GF diet) is a diet that eliminates foods containing gluten, a protein composite found in wheat (including kamut and spelt), barley, rye and triticale.

Macrobiotic: A Macrobiotic regimen consists of eating grains as the main staple in addition to local vegetables, and avoiding highly processed or refined foods and most animal products.

Paleo: The Paleo Diet is an effort to eat like we used to back in the day. If a caveman couldn't eat it, neither can you. This means eating anything we would hunt or find, including meat, fish, nuts, leafy greens, regional veggies and seeds.

Pescetarian: Similar to a vegetarian but they include fish in their diet.

Raw: A raw diet contains only uncooked and unprocessed foods. People following a raw diet eat fruits, vegetables, nuts and some grains.

Vegan: If someone is vegan they consume no animal flesh, including red meat, poultry or fish, or products that have come from an animal, such as eggs, milk or any dairy products.

Vegetarian: Vegetarians consume no meat – including red meat, poultry or fish – but may include eggs and dairy products as part of their diet.

RECIPES

Please note the following general points, which apply to all the recipes.

- All the recipes use standard UK/US spoon measures: 1 teaspoon (tsp) = 5 ml; 1 tablespoon (tbsp) = 15 ml. Note that in Australia 1 tsp = 5 ml, but 1 tbsp = 20 ml, so take care when measuring. All spoonfuls should be level.

- A handful is equal to about 8 oz/250 ml/1 cup.

- All eggs and produce are medium in size, unless a recipe states otherwise.

- Wash all produce before juicing, blending or cooking it.

- If you are unsure how to prepare a fruit or vegetable for juicing, check out our guide on page 19.

- Please note that the nutrition information for juices in particular is just an estimate. The actual calories and nutritional content will vary based on the size of your produce and the efficiency of your juicer.

- If using canned foods, such as beans or tomatoes, some authorities (such as the US Food and Drug Administration) advise against cans where the inside is coated with Biphenol-A (BPA). The same goes for plastic storage containers and bottles made with this chemical. Some research studies have linked BPA to breast cancer and diabetes, as well as to hyperactivity, aggression and depression in children.

Key

Colour Try to drink a variety of colours. Substitute like colour for like colour on a Reboot plan.

Season The ideal season in the UK for one or more key items in this recipe to help you get produce at its best.

R Appropriate for a Reboot (which all recipes in this book are except for some of the pulp recipes).

⏱ This is a quick and easy item to make, using few ingredients and no elaborate preparation.

🏃 Great for post-workout – or if it's a juice, even during your workout.

✚ Especially helpful if you have one or more of the listed health conditions.

Juices

All juices make 16–18fl oz/500ml but yield will vary based on the size of your produce and efficiency of your juicer.

These recipes are for a juicer (separates the juice from the pulp), alternatively you can use a blender plus a nut milk bag. For the difference between juicing and blending, see page 40.

Autumn Harvest

Orange

Autumn

R ⊙ 🏃

✚ cancer, arthritis, gout, allergies, migraines, inflammation/pain,
auto-immune conditions, thyroid, vision, skin, immunity

Nutrition per serving: 216 kCal; 903 kJ; 3 g protein; 49 g
carbohydrates; 1 g fat; 0 g saturated fat; 0 g fibre; 18 g sugar;
58 mg salt

1 butternut squash

1–2 red apples

1 tbsp ground cinnamon

1in/2.5cm piece of fresh root ginger

Call for Fall
Orange

Summer/Autumn

R 🏃

✚ Heart disease, stroke, high cholesterol, allergies, migraines, thyroid, weight loss/obesity, vision, skin, immunity

Nutrition per serving: 172 kCal; 720 kJ; 3 g protein; 39 g carbohydrates; 1 g fat; 0 g saturated fat; 3 g fibre; 25 g sugar; 52 mg salt

2 carrots

1½ apples

½ lemon

4 leaves romaine (cos) lettuce

5 strawberries

Celebration Grape Vino

Purple

Summer/Autumn

R ⋏

✚ Heart disease, cancer, arthritis, thyroid, GI, liver

Nutrition per serving: 248 kCal; 1038 kJ; 7 g protein; 53 g carbohydrates; 1 g fat; 0 g saturated fat; 5 g fibre; 38 g sugar; 56 mg salt

½ fennel bulb

½ head of red cabbage

2 large handfuls of grapes

1 green apple

Citrus Winter Warmer

Red

Winter

R 🏃

✚ Heart disease, stroke, high cholesterol, cancer, auto-immune
conditions, thyroid, skin, immunity, GI, liver

Nutrition per serving: 232 kCal; 971 kJ; 5 g protein; 52 g
carbohydrates; 1 g fat; 0 g saturated fat; 3 g fibre; 29 g sugar;
48 mg salt

2 blood or regular oranges

½ ruby grapefruit

1 beetroot (beet)

1 sweet potato

½ lemon

1in/2.5cm piece of fresh ginger root

Clean Green Bean

Green

Summer

R

+ stroke, diabetes, osteoporosis, thyroid, weight loss/obesity, skin, GI

Nutrition per serving: 123 kCal; 515 kJ; 5 g protein; 24 g carbohydrates; 1 g fat; 0 g saturated fat; 1 g fibre; 10 g sugar; 24 mg salt

2 large handfuls of green beans
  (about 7oz/200g)

1 large handful of spinach leaves
  (about 7oz/200g)

2 cucumbers

1 lemon

Cooling Summer

Red

Summer

R ◔

✚ thyroid, skin

Nutrition per serving: 239 kCal; 1000 kJ; 5 g protein; 51 g
carbohydrates; 2 g fat; 0 g saturated fat; 2 g fibre; 33 g sugar;
23 mg salt

14oz/450g/1 cup strawberries

2 apples

2 courgettes (zucchinis)

2 celery sticks

Dark & Stormy

Purple

Summer/Autumn

R 🏃

✚ Heart disease, high cholesterol, diabetes, cancer, osteoporosis, arthritis, inflammation/pain, weight loss/obesity, immunity, GI, liver, menstrual/PMS/menopause/PCOS

Nutrition per serving: 121 kCal; 506 kJ; 6 g protein; 21 g carbohydrates; 1 g fat; 0 g saturated fat; 2 g fibre; 6 g sugar; 63 mg salt

8 red kale (Tuscan cabbage) leaves

1 large beetroot (beet)

1 bunch of fresh parsley

2 celery sticks

1 lemon

Deep Dive Green

Green

Summer

R 🏃

✚ Heart disease, diabetes, osteoporosis, vision, immunity, memory, liver, menstrual/PMS/menopause/PCOS

Nutrition per serving: 105 kCal; 439 kJ; 6 g protein; 18 g carbohydrates; 1 g fat; 0 g saturated fat; 1 g fibre; 6 g sugar; 66 mg salt

4 kale (Tuscan cabbage) leaves

2 romaine (cos) leaves

1 small handful of spinach leaves

1 small handful of fresh parsley

4 celery sticks

½ cucumber

½ courgette (zucchini)

1 lime

1in/2.5cm piece of fresh root ginger

Divine Dreamsicle

Orange

Autumn/Spring

R ⚡

✚ Heart disease, stroke, high cholesterol, cancer, arthritis,
allergies, migraines, inflammation/pain, auto-immune
conditions, thyroid, vision, skin, immunity

Nutrition per serving: 237 kCal; 992 kJ; 5 g protein; 53 g
carbohydrates; 1 g fat; 0 g saturated fat; 4 g fibre; 34 g sugar;
47 mg salt

1 apple

¼ pineapple

1 sweet potato

4–6 carrots

Extreme Green

Green

Summer/Autumn

R

✚ Heart disease, stroke, high cholesterol, cancer, osteoporosis, arthritis, inflammation/pain, vision, skin, immunity, liver

Nutrition per serving: 220 kCal; 920 kJ; 5 g protein; 47 g carbohydrates; 1 g fat; 0 g saturated fat; 1 g fibre; 32 g sugar; 13 mg salt

½ cucumber

½ courgette (zucchini)

1 small handful of fresh parsley

4 kale (Tuscan cabbage) leaves

3 celery sticks

1 handful of green grapes

1 apple

¼ lime

Fall Back to Summer
Orange

Summer/Autumn

R 🏃

✚ stroke, cancer, arthritis, gout, allergies, migraines,
inflammation/pain, auto-immune conditions, thyroid, vision,
skin, immunity

Nutrition per serving: 222 kCal; 929 kJ; 3 g protein; 51 g
carbohydrates; 1 g fat; 0 g saturated fat; 1 g fibre; 28 g sugar;
50 mg salt

1 sweet potato

½ cantaloupe (rockmelon)

1 pear

dash of ground cinnamon

1in/2.5cm piece of fresh root ginger

Fennel & Spice & Everything Nice

Red

Summer/Autumn

R

+ Heart disease, stroke, high cholesterol, diabetes, cancer, osteoporosis, arthritis, gout, allergies, migraines, inflammation/pain, auto-immune conditions, weight loss/obesity, vision, skin, immunity, liver, menstrual/PMS/menopause/PCOS

Nutrition per serving: 231 kCal; 891 kJ; 7 g protein; 42 g carbohydrates; 2 g fat; 0 g saturated fat; 4 g fibre; 14 g sugar; 60 mg salt

½ fennel bulb

4 medium carrots

2 sweet red (bell) peppers (capsicum)

6–8 kale (Tuscan cabbage) leaves

2in/5cm piece of fresh root ginger

Field of Green Dreams
Green

Autumn/Winter

R

✚ Heart disease, stroke, cancer, osteoporosis, migraines, auto-
immune conditions, weight loss/obesity, vision, skin, immunity

Nutrition per serving: 146 kCal; 611 kJ; 4 g protein; 31 g
carbohydrates; 1 g fat; 0 g saturated fat; 1 g fibre; 17 g sugar;
44 mg salt

1 large handful of spinach leaves

1 cucumber

1 small handful of fresh parsley

1 apple

1 lime

Giant Green Peach
Orange

Summary

R

➕ Heart disease, stroke, diabetes, cancer, osteoporosis, arthritis, gout, allergies, migraines, inflammation/pain, auto-immune conditions, weight loss/obesity, vision, skin, immunity, liver, menstrual/PMS/menopause/PCOS

Nutrition per serving: 105 kCal; 439 kJ; 3 g protein; 21 g carbohydrates; 1 g fat; 0 g saturated fat; 2 g fibre; 12 g sugar; 55 mg salt

1 peach

4 kale (Tuscan cabbage) leaves

2 carrots

1in/2.5cm piece of fresh root ginger

Heart Beet

Purple

Autumn

R

✚ Heart disease, stroke, high cholesterol, diabetes, cancer, osteoporosis, arthritis, gout, weight loss/obesity, vision, skin, immunity, GI, liver, menstrual/PMS/menopause/PCOS, gall bladder

Nutrition per serving: 248 kCal; 1038 kJ; 7 g protein; 53 g carbohydrates; 1 g fat; 0 g saturated fat; 2 g fibre; 34 g sugar; 66 mg salt

1 beetroot (beet)

2 rainbow chard (silverbeet) leaves

2 celery sticks

1 broccoli stem

1 large handful of fresh basil

1 lemon

2 green apples

Heart Warmer
Purple

Autumn

R ⚡

✚ Heart disease, stroke, high cholesterol, cancer, allergies, migraines, vision, immunity, memory, GI, liver

Nutrition per serving: 232 kCal; 971 kJ; 4 g protein; 53 g carbohydrates; 1 g fat; 0 g saturated fat; 4 g fibre; 33 g sugar; 55 mg salt

2 beetroots (beets) and their leaves

4 chard (silverbeet) leaves

2 carrots

2 apples

1in/2.5cm piece of fresh root ginger

Heartbreak Hill

Red

Winter

R 🏃

✚ Heart disease, stroke, high cholesterol, arthritis, inflammation/
pain, thyroid, immunity, GI, liver

Nutrition per serving: 157 kCal; 657 kJ; 4 g protein; 34 g
carbohydrates; 1 g fat; 0 g saturated fat; 5 g fibre; 24 g sugar;
34 mg salt

2 small beetroots (beets)

2 oranges

2in/5cm slice of fresh root ginger

2 romaine lettuce leaves

Heavenly Honeydew

Green

Summer

R 🏃

✚ diabetes, osteoporosis, thyroid, weight loss/obesity, skin, menstrual/PMS/menopause/PCOS

Nutrition per serving: 98 kCal; 410 kJ; 3 g protein; 19 g carbohydrates; 1 g fat; 0 g saturated fat; 1 g fibre; 11 g sugar; 64 mg salt

1 handful of spinach leaves

¼ honeydew melon

1 cucumber

1 lemon

Holly Jolly

Purple

Winter

R 🏃

✚ Heart disease, stroke, cancer, inflammation/pain, immunity, memory, GI, liver

Nutrition per serving: 249 kCal; 1042 kJ; 7 g protein; 51 g carbohydrates; 2 g fat; 0 g saturated fat; 5 g fibre; 36 g sugar; 51 mg salt

¼ head of red cabbage

5 small or 2 medium-sized beetroots (beets)

3 clementines or 1 orange

115g/½ cup pomegranate seeds

2 large romaine lettuce leaves

Joe's Mean Green

Green

Winter

R

✚ Heart disease, high cholesterol, cancer, osteoporosis, arthritis, migraines, inflammation/pain, auto-immune conditions, weight loss/obesity, vision, skin, immunity, liver

Nutrition per serving: 225 kCal; 941 kJ; 5 g protein; 48 g carbohydrates; 1 g fat; 0 g saturated fat; 2 g fibre; 30 g sugar; 57 mg salt

8 kale (Tuscan cabbage) leaves

1 cucumber

4 celery sticks

2 apples

½ lemon

1in/2.5cm piece of fresh root ginger

Joyous Julius

Orange

Summer/Autumn

R ⏱

✚ Heart disease, stroke, high cholesterol, cancer, arthritis, allergies, migraines, inflammation/pain, auto-immune conditions, thyroid, vision, skin, immunity

Nutrition per serving: 159 kCal; 665 kJ; 4 g protein; 34 g carbohydrates; 1 g fat; 0 g saturated fat; 4 g fibre; 21 g sugar; 59 mg salt

1 sweet orange (bell) pepper (capsicum)

1 orange

5 carrots

1 large handful of spinach leaves

Kumquat Kooler

Orange

Winter

R ⏲

✚ Heart disease, stroke, cancer, arthritis, gout, allergies, inflammation/pain, thyroid, vision, skin, immunity

Nutrition per serving: 181 kCal; 757 kJ; 4 g protein; 38 g carbohydrates; 1 g fat; 0 g saturated fat; 4 g fibre; 20 g sugar; 59 mg salt

6 kumquats

1 sweet orange (bell) pepper (capsicum)

8 carrots

1in/2.5cm piece of fresh root ginger

Lean Green Pineapple

Green

Spring

R ⏲

✚ Heart disease, diabetes, cancer, osteoporosis, arthritis, gout, inflammation/pain, auto-immune conditions, thyroid

Nutrition per serving: 160 kCal; 669 kJ; 7 g protein; 31 g carbohydrates; 1 g fat; 0 g saturated fat; 1 g fibre; 16 g sugar; 55 mg salt

2 large handfuls of spinach leaves (about 12oz/340g)

¼ pineapple

1 lemon

Lime Dance

Green

Spring

R

✚ diabetes, osteoporosis, migraines, inflammation/pain, weight
loss/obesity, vision, skin, immunity, GI, liver, menstrual/PMS/
menopause/PCOS

Nutrition per serving: 157 kCal; 657 kJ; 3 g protein; 34 g
carbohydrates; 1 g fat; 0 g saturated fat; 4 g fibre; 19 g sugar;
50 mg salt

¼ pineapple

1 cucumber

1 lime

1 handful of fresh coriander (cilantro)

1 large handful of dandelion greens

Love Your Broccoli
Orange

Autumn

R ⊘

✚ stroke, cancer, allergies, migraines, vision, skin, immunity

Nutrition per serving: 120 kCal; 502 kJ; 5 g protein; 24 g carbohydrates; 1 g fat; 0 g saturated fat; 3 g fibre; 11 g sugar; 60 mg salt

4 carrots

6 strawberries

1 broccoli stem

Lucky Leprechaun
Red

Summer/Autumn

R

✚ diabetes, cancer, allergies, migraines, auto-immune
conditions, weight loss/obesity, vision, skin, immunity, GI, liver,
menstrual/PMS/menopause/PCOS, gall bladder

Nutrition per serving: 233 kCal; 975 kJ; 8 g protein; 46 g
carbohydrates; 2 g fat; 0 g saturated fat; 4 g fibre; 16 g sugar;
45 mg salt

5 medium–large carrots

1 medium tomato

½ head of broccoli

1 handful of fresh parsley

1 lime

2in/5cm piece of fresh root ginger

Mint to Be Green

Green

Summer

R

✚ Heart disease, diabetes, arthritis, inflammation/pain, thyroid, weight loss/obesity, skin, menstrual/PMS/menopause/PCOS

Nutrition per serving: 100 kCal; 418 kJ; 3 g protein; 20 g carbohydrates; 1 g fat; 0 g saturated fat; 0 g fibre; 9 g sugar; 34 mg salt

¼ honeydew melon

2 celery sticks

½ cucumber

½ lime

1 handful of fresh mint

Morning OJ

Orange

Summer/Autumn

R

✚ stroke, diabetes, cancer, arthritis, allergies, migraines, inflammation/pain, auto-immune conditions, thyroid, weight loss/obesity, vision, skin, immunity, menstrual/PMS/Menopause/PCOS

Nutrition per serving: 118 kCal; 494 kJ; 3 g protein; 25 g carbohydrates; 1 g fat; 0 g saturated fat; 2 g fibre; 10 g sugar; 51 mg salt

1 sweet orange (bell) pepper (capsicum)

1 sweet yellow (bell) pepper (capsicum)

1 large carrot

½ green apple

½ lemon

Morning Red Riser

Red

Summer/Autumn

R 🏃

✚ cancer, migraines, thyroid, vision, skin, immunity, GI

Nutrition per serving: 184 kCal; 770 kJ; 4 g protein; 38 g carbohydrates; 2 g fat; 0 g saturated fat; 2 g fibre; 28 g sugar; 51 mg salt

1 beetroot (beet)

1 purple carrot (or orange carrot)

12 strawberries

2 oranges

2 celery sticks

New Beginnings
Purple

Summer/Autumn

R ⚹

✚ stroke, thyroid, vision, skin, immunity, GI, liver

Nutrition per serving: 183 kCal; 766 kJ; 5 g protein; 38 g
carbohydrates; 1 g fat; 0 g saturated fat; 4 g fibre; 22 g sugar;
64 mg salt

4 large carrots

2 medium beetroots (beets)

2 medium sweet red (bell) peppers
(capsicum)

1in/2.5cm piece of fresh root ginger

Not Too Sweet Cucumber Melon Juice

Green

Summer

R ⊙ 🏃

✚ Heart disease, diabetes, auto-immune conditions, thyroid,
weight loss/obesity, skin, menstrual/PMS/menopause/PCOS

Nutrition per serving: 118 kCal; 494 kJ; 4 g protein; 24 g
carbohydrates; 1 g fat; 0 g saturated fat; 0 g fibre; 14 g sugar;
38 mg salt

2 large cucumbers

¼ honeydew melon

3 celery sticks

Passionate Plum

Green

Summer/Autumn

R ⊘ ⃗

✚ Heart disease, arthritis, thyroid, weight loss/obesity, skin, memory

Nutrition per serving: 98 kCal; 410 kJ; 2 g protein; 18 g carbohydrates; 2 g fat; 0 g saturated fat; 1 g fibre; 14 g sugar; 50 mg salt

1 cucumber

5 celery sticks

1–2 plums

Picnic Party
Green

Summer

R ⫪

✚ arthritis, gout, allergies, immunity, GI, liver

Nutrition per serving: 222 kCal; 929 kJ; 7 g protein; 46 g carbohydrates; 1 g fat; 0 g saturated fat; 5 g fibre; 26 g sugar; 50 mg salt

1 yellow beetroot (beet)

½ grapefruit

1 summer squash

½ cucumber

¼ head of green cabbage

1 apple (or pear)

1 small handful of fresh mint

Pineapple Power

Green

Spring

R ⊙ ⃛

✚ Heart disease, stroke, high cholesterol, diabetes, cancer, osteoporosis, arthritis, migraines, inflammation/pain, weight loss/obesity, vision, skin, immunity, GI, liver, menstrual/PMS/menopause/PCOS, gall bladder

Nutrition per serving: 133 kCal; 556 kJ; 4 g protein; 28 g carbohydrates; 1 g fat; 0 g saturated fat; 1 g fibre; 16 g sugar; 51 mg salt

¼ pineapple

1 large handful of watercress

4–6 kale (Tuscan cabbage) leaves

2 celery sticks

Pink Lemonade

Red

Summer

R

+ stroke, cancer, inflammation/pain, auto-immune conditions, skin, immunity, GI, liver, gall bladder

Nutrition per serving: 241 kCal; 1008 kJ; 7 g protein; 51 g carbohydrates; 1 g fat; 0 g saturated fat; 4 g fibre; 29 g sugar; 52 mg salt

2 pears

1 lemon

¼ head of green cabbage

1 large handful of spinach leaves

1 small handful of fresh mint

12 strawberries

Piping Hot Pepper

Red

Summer/Autumn

R

+ Heart disease, stroke, high cholesterol, diabetes, cancer, arthritis, inflammation/pain, auto-immune conditions, thyroid, weight loss/obesity, vision, skin, immunity, GI, menstrual/PMS/menopause/PCOS

Nutrition per serving: 105 kCal; 439 kJ; 3 g protein; 21 g carbohydrates; 1 g fat; 0 g saturated fat; 1 g fibre; 10 g sugar; 44 mg salt

1 sweet green (bell) pepper (capsicum)

1 sweet yellow (bell) pepper (capsicum)

1 sweet red (bell) pepper (capsicum)

1 chilli pepper (jalapeño) (optional)

2 celery sticks

1 lime

1 small handful of fresh coriander (cilantro)

Purest Green

Green

Winter

R

✚ Heart disease, osteoporosis, weight loss/obesity, skin, immunity, memory, GI, gall bladder

Nutrition per serving: 209 kCal; 874 kJ; 8 g protein; 42 g carbohydrates; 1 g fat; 0 g saturated fat; 4 g fibre; 14 g sugar; 52 mg salt

8 kale (Tuscan cabbage) leaves

1 cucumber

¼ head of cabbage

4 celery sticks

1 orange

1 lime

Rainbow Bright
Green

Autumn/Winter

R ⏱

➕ Heart disease, stroke, high cholesterol, osteoporosis, allergies, migraines, auto-immune conditions, vision, skin, immunity, liver

Nutrition per serving: 241 kCal; 1008 kJ; 4 g protein; 53 g carbohydrates; 1 g fat; 0 g saturated fat; 4 g fibre; 33 g sugar; 54 mg salt

4 kale (Tuscan cabbage) leaves

3 celery sticks

4 carrots

2 apples

Skin Brightening

Green

Autumn/Winter

R ☉

✚ Heart disease, cancer, osteoporosis, allergies, skin, migraines, weight loss/obesity, immunity, GI, liver, gall bladder

Nutrition per serving: 265 kCal; 1109 kJ; 10 g protein; 52 g carbohydrates; 2 g fat; 0 g saturated fat; 5 g fibre; 27 g sugar; 64 mg salt

2 oranges

2 carrots

1 head of broccoli

2 celery sticks

Slim Grin

Green

Autumn

R ⊙

✚ Heart disease, migraines, thyroid, skin, immunity

Nutrition per serving: 245 kCal; 1025 kJ; 3 g protein; 57 g carbohydrates; 1 g fat; 0 g saturated fat; 2 g fibre; 35 g sugar; 64 mg salt

2 large green pears

1 handful of green grapes

1 large bunch of spinach leaves

1 cucumber

Spiced Sweet Potato
Orange

Winter

R ⚥

✚ stroke, cancer, allergies, migraines, auto-immune conditions, thyroid, vision, skin, immunity

Nutrition per serving: 146 kCal; 611 kJ; 3 g protein; 33 g carbohydrates; 1 g fat; 0 g saturated fat; 2 g fibre; 14 g sugar; 49 mg salt

1 large sweet potato

2 carrots

1 tangerine

¼ tsp ground cinnamon

dash of nutmeg

Springing High

Green

Spring

R 🏃

➕ Heart disease, cancer, osteoporosis, arthritis, gout, migraines, inflammation/pain, auto-immune conditions, weight loss/obesity, vision, skin, immunity, liver

Nutrition per serving: 241 kCal; 1008 kJ; 5 g protein; 52 g carbohydrates; 1 g fat; 0 g saturated fat; 2 g fibre; 26 g sugar; 53 mg salt

1 fennel bulb

6 kale (Tuscan cabbage) leaves

2 limes

2 apples

Summer Shine

Orange

Summer

R 🏃

✚ Heart disease, cancer, allergies, auto-immune conditions, thyroid, vision, skin

Nutrition per serving: 118 kCal; 495 kJ; 3 g protein; 25 g carbohydrates; 1 g fat; 0 g saturated fat; 2 g fibre; 16 g sugar; 104 mg salt

5 celery sticks

½ cucumber

1 large carrot

1 tomato

½ orange

½ peach

Sunny Green

Green

¼ pineapple

4 celery sticks

1 large bunch of romaine (cos) lettuce

1 handful of spinach leaves

1 lime

Sunny Pineapple

Yellow

Spring

R ⊙ 🏃

✚ arthritis, gout, migraines, inflammation/pain, auto-immune conditions, thyroid, skin

Nutrition per serving: 107 kCal; 448 kJ; 2 g protein; 23 g carbohydrates; 1 g fat; 0 g saturated fat; 1 g fibre; 16 g sugar; 46 mg salt

¼ pineapple

4 celery sticks

1in/2.5cm piece of fresh root ginger

Sweet & Sour

Green

Winter

R ⊙ 👟

✚ osteoporosis, arthritis, gout, thyroid, skin, immunity

Nutrition per serving: 138 kCal; 577 kJ; 3 g protein; 30 g carbohydrates; 1 g fat; 0 g saturated fat; 4 g fibre; 24 g sugar; 54 mg salt

2 large handfuls of spinach leaves (about 12oz/340g)

3 celery sticks

2 grapefruits

Sweet n' Tangy

Green

Summer/Autumn

R

✚ Heart disease, high cholesterol, cancer, osteoporosis, arthritis, inflammation/pain, weight loss/obesity, skin, liver

Nutrition per serving: 196 kCal; 820 kJ; 3 g protein; 44 g carbohydrates; 1 g fat; 0 g saturated fat; 2 g fibre; 23 g sugar; 68 mg salt

1 large radish

1 small apple

1 pear

½ fennel bulb

4 kale (Tuscan cabbage) leaves

Sweet Sage

Green

Winter

R

✚ Heart disease, stroke, high cholesterol, inflammation/pain, auto-immune conditions, weight loss/obesity, liver

Nutrition per serving: 155 kCal; 649 kJ; 3 g protein; 33 g carbohydrates; 1 g fat; 0 g saturated fat; 4 g fibre; 12 g sugar; 57 mg salt

½ lime

1 handful of fresh sage leaves

2 celery sticks

1–2 pears

¼ head of green cabbage

Trick-or-Treat

Orange

Autumn

R ⚡

✚ Heart disease, stroke, high cholesterol, diabetes, cancer, arthritis, gout, allergies, migraines, inflammation/pain, thyroid, vision, skin, immunity, menstrual/PMS/menopause/PCOS

Nutrition per serving: 162 kCal; 678 kJ; 3 g protein; 36 g carbohydrates; 1 g fat; 0 g saturated fat; 3 g fibre; 16 g sugar; 57 mg salt

1 sweet potato

1 orange

1 sweet orange (bell) pepper (capsicum)

1 carrot

dash of ground cinnamon

Tropical Mint
Yellow

Spring

R ☉ 🏃

➕ arthritis, gout, inflammation/pain, auto-immune conditions, thyroid, skin

Nutrition per serving: 219 kCal; 916 kJ; 4 g protein; 49 g carbohydrates; 1 g fat; 0 g saturated fat; 0 g fibre; 33 g sugar; 13 mg salt

½ pineapple

1 cucumber

1 large handful of fresh mint

1in/2.5cm piece of fresh root ginger

Turnip the Greens
Green

Autumn

R

✚ Heart disease, migraines, auto-immune conditions, thyroid, weight loss/obesity, vision, skin, immunity

Nutrition per serving: 180 kCal; 753 kJ; 4 g protein; 40 g carbohydrates; 1 g fat; 0 g saturated fat; 3 g fibre; 25 g sugar; 64 mg salt

1 large turnip

1 pear

½ cucumber

2 handfuls of spinach leaves

¼ cantaloupe (rockmelon)

1 large carrot

Warrior Princess
Red

Summer

R 🏃

✚ Heart disease, stroke, high cholesterol, cancer, inflammation/
pain, vision, skin, immunity, GI, liver

Nutrition per serving: 227 kCal; 950 kJ; 6 g protein; 49 g
carbohydrates; 1 g fat; 0 g saturated fat; 5 g fibre; 33 g sugar;
58 mg salt

½ head of red cabbage

½ small watermelon

2 oranges

½ fennel bulb

Watercress Wonder

Green

Spring

R ⊙ 🏃

✚ Heart disease, high cholesterol, cancer, arthritis, skin, liver, gall bladder

Nutrition per serving: 167 kCal; 699 kJ; 1 g protein; 39 g carbohydrates; 1 g fat; 0 g saturated fat; 1 g fibre; 26 g sugar; 46 mg salt

1 large bunch of watercress (7oz/200g)

2 green apples

1 lime

2 celery sticks

Workout to the Beet

Purple

Winter

R ☉ 🏃

✚ Heart disease, stroke, cancer, thyroid, weight loss/obesity, skin, memory, GI

Nutrition per serving: 201 kCal; 840 kJ; 6 g protein; 43 g carbohydrates; 1 g fat; 0 g saturated fat; 3 g fibre; 30 g sugar; 45 mg salt

3 small beetroots (beets)

1 cucumber

1 handful of spinach leaves

2 oranges

Coconut water juices

On Juice-only days, our Reboot plans call for drinking 16 oz of coconut water. For a more flavourful twist, try these juice additions (but these count as your daily coconut water intake, not juice!).

Run the fruits and vegetables through your juicer and then mix with the coconut water, plus ice if you prefer a colder drink.

COCONUT WATER

Coconut water is something I didn't have on my Reboot, but I wish I'd known about it. As my nutritionist team has developed the Reboot plans, coconut water is something they've added as an essential item.

Coconut water is an important source of electrolytes, which are ions that carry electricity including sodium, chloride, potassium and magnesium, and are essential for the normal functioning of our cells and organs. You lose electrolytes when you sweat and you replace them by drinking fluids.

Drinking electrolyte-rich fluids on a Reboot can help alleviate many of the side-effects commonly experienced in the first few days of the plan – feeling light-headed, dizziness, fatigue, headaches, foggy brain . . . They're also important if you have leg cramps, vomiting or diarrhoea.

But some Rebooters just don't like the taste of coconut water. If this sounds like you, I recommend mixing it with juice. So we've come up with a few special recipes for 'flavoured' coconut water just for you.

Mint Coconut Colada

Green

Spring/Summer

R ⊙ 🏃

✚ Heart disease, stroke, cancer, osteoporosis, gout,
inflammation/pain, auto-immune conditions, weight loss/
obesity, vision, immunity, GI

Nutrition per serving: 142 kCal; 594 kJ; 4 g protein; 29 g
carbohydrates; 1 g fat; 0 g saturated fat; 1 g fibre; 20 g sugar;
71 mg salt

¼ pineapple

2 celery sticks

1 small handful of fresh mint

8–16fl oz/225–450ml/1–2 cups coconut
water

Green Coconut Water

Green

Autumn

R 🏃

➕ Heart disease, diabetes, cancer, osteoporosis, inflammation/
pain, auto-immune conditions, weight loss/obesity, vision,
skin, immunity, memory, GI, liver, gall bladder

Nutrition per serving: 194 kCal; 812 kJ; 5 g protein; 40 g
carbohydrates; 1 g fat; 0 g saturated fat; 1 g fibre; 24 g sugar;
44 mg salt

4 kale (Tuscan cabbage) leaves

1 cucumber

1 celery stick

1 apple

8–16fl oz/225–450ml/1–2 cups coconut
water

Strawberry on the Vine Coconut Water

Green

Summer

R ☉ ⅄

✚ Heart disease, stroke, high cholesterol, diabetes, cancer, osteoporosis, gout, allergies, inflammation/pain, vision, skin, immunity, GI, menstrual/PMS/menopause/PCOS

Nutrition per serving: 105 kCal; 439 kJ; 4 g protein; 20 g carbohydrates; 1 g fat; 0 g saturated fat; 0 g fibre; 11 g sugar; 63 mg salt

8 strawberries

1 small handful of fresh mint

1 large handful of spinach leaves

8–16fl oz/225–450ml/1–2 cups coconut water

Sweet Lime Coconut Water

Orange

Autumn/Winter

R ☉ ⸸

✚ Heart disease, high cholesterol, diabetes, arthritis, gout, migraines, auto-immune conditions, weight loss/obesity, vision, skin, immunity, GI, liver, menstrual/PMS/menopause/PCOS, gall bladder

Nutrition per serving: 144 kCal; 602 kJ; 4 g protein; 31 g carbohydrates; 1 g fat; 0 g saturated fat; 1 g fibre; 12 g sugar; 70 mg salt

1 sweet potato

½ lime

8–16fl oz/225–450ml/1–2 cups coconut water

Smoothies

Remember a smoothie is made in a blender, not your juicer. (For the difference between juicing and blending see page 40.) For each of these recipes make the juice element and then simply put everything in your blender and whiz it up!

All smoothies make 16–18fl oz/500ml.

Berries & Beet

Summer

R ⊙ 🏃

✚ Heart disease, cancer, gout, inflammation/pain, auto-immune
conditions, vision, skin, immunity, liver

Nutrition per serving: 220kCal; 920kJ; 6g protein; 50g carbohydrates;
1.5g fat; 0g saturated fat; 13g fibre; 33g sugar; 340mg salt

8fl oz/225ml/1 cup coconut water

4oz/110g/1 cup raspberries, fresh or frozen

4oz/110g/1 cup cherries, fresh or frozen

4½oz/110g/1 cup strawberries, fresh or
frozen

1 tbsp goji berries (optional)

½–1 small beetroot (beet), peeled

½ small carrot

1 handful of ice (3–4 cubes)

Cucumber Melon

Summer

R

+ stroke, cancer, arthritis, gout, inflammation/pain, thyroid, weight loss/obesity, vision, skin, immunity, GI, menstrual/PMS/menopause/PCOS

Nutrition per serving: 120kCal; 502kJ; 3g protein; 30g carbohydrates; 0.5g fat; 0g saturated fat; 3g fibre; 24g sugar; 400mg salt

¼ honeydew melon

½ cucumber

1 celery stick

juice of ½ lime

pinch of sea salt (optional)

1 handful of ice (3–4 cubes)

Fire Engine Red

Autumn/Winter

R

✚ Heart disease, stroke, high cholesterol, cancer, osteoporosis,
arthritis, inflammation/pain, auto-immune conditions, thyroid,
vision, skin, immunity, liver, menstrual/PMS/menopause/PCOS

Nutrition per serving: 400kCal; 1672kJ; 10g protein; 89g
carbohydrates; 4g fat; 1g saturated fat; 19g fibre; 65g sugar;
490mg salt

8oz/230g/1 cup pomegranate seeds

2 tbsp goji berries (optional)

½ small beetroot (beet), peeled

13fl oz/375ml/1½ cups coconut water

Ginger Joy

Spring

R

✚ Heart disease, high cholesterol, diabetes, cancer, osteoporosis, arthritis, gout, allergies, migraines, inflammation/pain, auto-immune conditions, vision, GI, menstrual/PMS/menopause/PCOS

Nutrition per serving: 200kCal; 836kJ; 8g protein; 45g carbohydrates; 0.5g fat; 0g saturated fat; 12g fibre; 28g sugar; 330mg salt

1 cucumber

1 handful of spinach leaves

1 green apple, cored

1 handful of fresh parsley

1in/2.5cm piece of fresh root ginger

8fl oz/225ml/1 cup coconut water

Great Green Pear

R

✚ High cholesterol, thyroid, cancer, skin, GI, osteoporosis

Nutrition per serving: 413 kCal; 1728kJ; 6 g protein; 74 g
carbohydrates; 16 g fat; 2 g saturated fat; 22 g fibre; 38 g sugar;
62 mg salt

2 pears, juiced (and frozen into ice cubes,
optional)

2 handfuls spinach

½ cucumber, juiced

½ avocado

1-in/2.5cm lemongrass stalk, chopped
(remove outer layer)

1 handful of ice (3–4 cubes)

Honey I Dew

Summer

R ⏱

✚ Heart disease, stroke, arthritis, gout, migraines, inflammation/
pain, immunity, GI, menstrual/PMS/menopause/PCOS

Nutrition per serving: 150kCal; 627kJ; 3g protein; 35g
carbohydrates; 0g fat; 0g saturated fat; 9g fibre; 22g sugar; 400mg
salt

3 handfuls of spinach leaves
(about 4oz/110g)

¼ honeydew melon, rind removed
(about 7oz/200g)

8fl oz/225ml/1 cup coconut water

1 handful of ice (3–4 cubes)

Pink Pom-Pom

Spring/Summer/Autumn

R

✚ Heart disease, diabetes, cancer, osteoporosis, arthritis, gout, allergies, migraines, inflammation/pain, vision, immunity, memory, liver

Nutrition per serving: 350kCal; 1463kJ; 9g protein; 78g carbohydrates; 4g fat; 1g saturated fat; 18g fibre; 57g sugar; 280mg salt

8oz/230g/1 cup pomegranate seeds

1 orange, peeled

8fl oz/225ml/1 cup coconut water

1 large handful of spinach leaves

Put the Lime in the Coconut

Spring

R

✚ Heart disease, stroke, high cholesterol, diabetes, cancer, gout, vision, immunity, memory, GI, menstrual/PMS/menopause/PCOS

Nutrition per serving: 140kCal; 585kJ; 4g protein; 34g carbohydrates; 1g fat; 0.5g saturated fat; 7g fibre; 16g sugar; 330mg salt

juice of 1 lime

8fl oz/225ml/1 cup coconut water

½ banana

2 handfuls of spinach leaves

1 handful of ice (3–4 cubes)

Raz-Avocado

Summer

R

✚ Heart disease, stroke, high cholesterol, diabetes, cancer, arthritis, gout, allergies, thyroid, vision, skin, immunity, memory

Nutrition per serving: 320kCal; 1338kJ; 7g protein; 42g carbohydrates; 16g fat; 2.5g saturated fat; 20g fibre; 14g sugar; 270mg salt

5oz/150g/1¼ cups raspberries, fresh or frozen

7oz/200g/1½ cups strawberries, fresh or frozen

½ avocado

1 handful of rocket (arugula)

8fl oz/225ml/1 cup coconut water

Sweet Basil

Summer

R

✛ Heart disease, high cholesterol, diabetes, cancer, osteoporosis, inflammation/pain, thyroid, vision, immunity, memory

Nutrition per serving: 200kCal; 836kJ; 8g protein; 45g carbohydrates; 0.5g fat; 0g saturated fat; 8g fibre; 32g sugar; 270mg salt

¼ pineapple, cored and skin removed

1 cucumber

1 handful of fresh basil

8fl oz/225ml/1 cup coconut water

1 handful of ice (3–4 cubes)

Sweet Bunny Love

Autumn/Winter

R

✚ Stroke, vision, skin, immunity , exercise, migraine, allergy, high BP, thyroid

Nutrition per serving: 321 kCal; 1343kJ; 6 g protein; 78 g carbohydrates; 1 g fat; 0 g saturated fat; 17 g fibre; 33 g sugar; 212 mg salt

1 large sweet potato, juiced (and frozen into ice cubes, optional)

4 carrots, juiced

1 banana

1 date, pitted

Ice, optional

Pinch of cinnamon

Salads

Guacamole Over Greens

Summer

R ☉ 🏃

➕ diabetes, cancer, migraines, inflammation/pain, weight loss/
obesity, vision, skin, memory, GI, liver, menstrual/PMS/
menopause/PCOS, gall bladder

Serves 4

Nutrition per serving: 160kCal; 669kJ; 2g protein; 10g
carbohydrates; 14g fat; 2g saturated fat; 8g fibre; 2g sugar; 20mg
salt

2 ripe avocados, diced

1 plum tomato, seeded and diced

¼ medium red onion, finely diced

½ chilli pepper (jalapeño), deseeded and
minced

juice of ½ lime

2 tbsp fresh coriander (cilantro), chopped

¼ tsp ground cumin

1 dash cayenne pepper (or more if you prefer a lot of heat)

kosher salt, to taste

2 large handfuls of spinach leaves

1 To make the guacamole, put all the ingredients except the spinach in a bowl and mix using a potato masher or fork. Season to taste, then spoon the guacamole over the spinach and serve.

2 To store the guacamole place in an airtight container. Cover with plastic wrap, pressing the plastic wrap on top of the guacamole, sealing out the air, then put on the container lid. This will prevent discolouration of the avocado due to oxidation.

Fresh Fennel and Avocado Salad

Summer

R

✚ Heart disease, stroke, high cholesterol, diabetes, cancer, arthritis, gout, migraines, inflammation/pain, vision, immunity, memory, GI

Serves 1

Nutrition per serving: 430kCal; 1797kJ; 9g protein; 43g carbohydrates; 29g fat; 4g saturated fat; 17g fibre; 18g sugar; 115mg salt

½ orange

½ avocado

6 leaves cos (romaine) lettuce

¼ of a head of red cabbage, thinly sliced

¼ of a fennel bulb

For the dressing (makes enough for 4 servings)

1 handful of fresh basil leaves

1 garlic clove, chopped

2 tsp honey (optional)

4 tbsp olive oil

juice from ½ lemon

1 tbsp apple cider vinegar

sea salt and freshly ground pepper, to taste

1 Peel the orange and separate into sections, removing the white pith.

2 Cut the avocado in half, remove the flesh with a spoon then slice. Put the other half, with the pit in it, in the refrigerator for use in another meal.

3 Next make the dressing. Place the basil leaves in a blender or food processor with the garlic, then add the honey, olive oil, lemon juice, vinegar and salt and pepper. Blend until smooth.

4 Chop the lettuce and transfer to a bowl, then add the cabbage, fennel, orange and avocado to the bowl and mix well.

5 Toss about 2 tbsp of dressing with the lettuce leaves. Store the remaining dressing in the refrigerator up to 5 days.

Sweet Mango, Avocado and Tomato Salad

Summary

R

✚ Heart disease, stroke, high cholesterol, cancer, gout, migraines, inflammation/pain, auto-immune conditions, thyroid, vision, skin, immunity, memory, gall bladder

Serves 1

Nutrition per serving: 280kCal; 1170kJ; 3g protein; 32g carbohydrates; 18g fat; 2.5g saturated fat; 8g fibre; 23g sugar; 10mg salt

½ avocado, cut into chunks

½ mango, cut into chunks

4oz/110g/½ cup cherry tomatoes, halved

1 tbsp olive oil

1 tbsp lemon juice

1 garlic clove, minced

½ tbsp raw honey (optional)

sea salt and freshly ground pepper, to taste

1 Put the avocado, mango and cherry tomatoes into a large bowl.

2 In a separate bowl, combine the olive oil, lemon juice, garlic, honey (if using) and salt and pepper and stir until evenly mixed. Pour this dressing over the salad and toss well.

3 Store the salad in the fridge for 1 hour or longer before serving.

Hail to Kale Salad

Summer

R

+ Heart disease, stroke, high cholesterol, diabetes, cancer, osteoporosis, allergies, auto-immune conditions, weight loss/obesity, vision, skin, immunity, GI, liver

Serves 4

Nutrition per serving: 370kCal; 1547kJ; 6g protein; 40g carbohydrates; 23g fat; 3g saturated fat; 9 fibre; 22g sugar; 70mg salt

1 large head of kale (Tuscan cabbage), leaves only (save stems for juicing)

½ red onion, chopped

2 carrots, peeled and cut into thin circles

1 handful dried cranberries or blueberries

1 sweet red (bell) pepper (capsicum), deseeded and chopped

1 cucumber, sliced and quartered

1 avocado, cubed

13oz/370g/2½ cups cherry tomatoes (or other variety), halved

1 large handful of goji berries (optional)

4 tbsp olive oil

4 tbsp lemon juice

1 Rip the kale leaves into bite-size pieces then add to large salad bowl. Add all the vegetables, avocado, and berries. Mix well.

2 Combine the olive oil and lemon juice in a small bowl, then pour over the salad and toss the dressing through until thoroughly combined.

3 Place in the refrigerator to 'marinate' for 10–15 minutes before serving.

Chopped Cranberry & Greens Salad

Autumn/Winter

R

✚ diabetes, osteoporosis, gout, allergies, inflammation/pain, thyroid, vision, skin, immunity, memory, menstrual/PMS/menopause/PCOS, gall bladder

Serves 4

Nutrition per serving: 90kCal; 376kJ; 2g protein; 23g carbohydrates; 0g fat; 0g saturated fat; 5g fibre; 14g sugar; 10mg salt

> 1 bunch/16 leaves of spring (collard) greens (save the stems for your next green juice)
>
> 1 orange
>
> 1 apple (honeycrisp or other sweet variety works best)
>
> 7oz/200g/2 cups fresh or frozen cranberries
>
> 1 tbsp honey (optional)

1 Remove the collard green stems from the leaves, chop the leaves and place in a bowl.

2 Zest the orange, then peel and juice it with the apple.

3 Place the cranberries and honey (if using) in a food processor and pulse for a coarse chop adding the orange/apple juice in small batches.

4 Pour the dressing over the greens, sprinkle the orange zest over the salad, then serve immediately.

Roasted Carrot & Avocado Salad

Summer

R

✚ Heart disease, stroke, high cholesterol, arthritis, migraines, vision, skin, memory, GI, liver, menstrual/PMS/menopause/ PCOS, gall bladder

Serves 2

Nutrition per serving: 360kCal; 1505kJ; 6g protein; 27g carbohydrates; 28g fat; 4g saturated fat; 11g fibre; 8g sugar; 110mg salt

4 large carrots, cut lengthwise into quarters

2 tbsp olive oil

1 tbsp ground cumin

1 tsp dried red pepper flakes

1 avocado, sliced

juice of 1 lemon

3oz/90g/½ cup rocket (arugula)

1 bunch of spinach leaves

sea salt and freshly ground pepper, to taste

1 Preheat the oven to 190°C/375°F/gas 5. Place the carrots in a mixing bowl and add ½–1 tbsp olive oil, cumin, red pepper flakes, salt and pepper and toss until the carrots are evenly coated.

2 Spread the carrots out on a roasting pan and roast in the oven for 25–30 minutes until browned. Give the carrots a stir halfway through.

3 Next prepare the simple lemon dressing by mixing the lemon juice with the remaining olive oil and salt and pepper to taste.

4 Remove the carrots from the oven, combine with the greens and avocado and toss with the dressing. Serve and enjoy!

Wilted Kale and Summer Squash Salad with Parsley Gremolata

Summer

R

✚ Heart disease, stroke, high cholesterol, diabetes, cancer, osteoporosis, allergies, inflammation/pain, auto-immune conditions, weight loss/obesity, skin, immunity, memory, liver, gall bladder

Serves 4

Nutrition per serving: 140kCal; 585kJ; 10g protein; 29g carbohydrates; 2g fat; 0g saturated fat; 7g fibre; 7g sugar; 105mg salt

- 1 head of kale (Tuscan cabbage), stems removed, leaves roughly chopped

- 1 large yellow squash, cut into circles or half moons

- 1 large courgette (zucchini), cut into circles or half moons

- 2 garlic cloves, minced

- 2 big handfuls of fresh parsley, chopped

- juice of 1 lemon

- sea salt and freshly ground pepper

1 Place the kale leaves in a large pan with a small amount of water, cover and steam until wilted, about 3–5 minutes.

2 Add the squash and courgette to the pan and cook over a medium heat until the squash is just tender, about 5–7 minutes. Transfer to a bowl.

3 Mix together the garlic, parsley, lemon juice and salt.

4 Dress the kale and squash with the parsley sauce and serve warm or at room temperature.

Avocado Caprese Salad

Summer

R

+ Heart disease, stroke, high cholesterol, diabetes, cancer, arthritis, gout, migraines, inflammation/pain, thyroid, vision, skin, immunity, memory, menstrual/PMS/menopause/PCOS

Serves 2 as a light meal, 4 as an appetizer

Nutrition per serving: 240kCal; 1003kJ; 4g protein; 16g carbohydrates; 20g fat; 3g saturated fat; 10g fibre; 6g sugar; 20mg salt

2 large heirloom tomatoes (or any variety if heirloom aren't available)

½ avocado

8–16 fresh basil leaves

2 tbsp olive oil

2 tbsp balsamic vinegar, to taste

dash of Himalayan salt and freshly ground pepper, to taste

1 Wash the tomatoes well and cut off the ends, then slice each one into four thick slices. Slice the avocado, then assemble the tomato slices on a plate and top with the avocado.

2 Add 1–2 basil leaves to each tomato, then drizzle

with olive oil and balsamic vinegar and sprinkle a dash of Himalayan salt and pepper over.

3 Serve as an appetizer or a light meal.

Evergreen Salad

Winter

R ◷

✚ Heart disease, stroke, high cholesterol, cancer, osteoporosis, arthritis, migraines, auto-immune conditions, vision, immunity, memory, liver, gall bladder

Serves 2

Nutrition per serving: 200kCal; 836kJ; 5g protein; 30g carbohydrates; 8g fat; 1g saturated fat; 9g fibre; 14g sugar; 110mg salt

4 kale (Tuscan cabbage) leaves

4 large handfuls of spinach leaves

6 kumquats or clementines

4oz/110g /½ cup pomegranate seeds

1 tbsp olive oil

2 tbsp balsamic vinegar

1 Remove the kale leaves from the stem and tear into small bite-size pieces. Toss with the spinach in a large bowl to combine.

2 Slice the kumquats into thin circles, and add to the bowl along with the pomegranate seeds.

3 Combine the olive oil and balsamic vinegar in

a small bowl and stir. Pour over the salad and toss to coat the leaves. Let sit in the fridge for at least 15 minutes so the salad wilts a bit.

4 Serve on 2 plates and enjoy!

Colourful Cold Weather Salad

Autumn/Winter

R

+ cancer, arthritis, gout, inflammation/pain, vision, skin, immunity, memory, liver, menstrual/PMS/menopause/PCOS, gall bladder

Serves 4

Nutrition per serving: 210kCal; 878kJ; 7g protein; 32g carbohydrates; 8g fat; 1g saturated fat; 8g fibre; 8g sugar; 100mg salt

1 butternut squash, peeled and chopped

1 large beetroot (beet) or 2 small, chopped into small cubes

4oz/110g/1 cup Brussels sprouts, sliced in half

1 tbsp coconut oil

1 bunch of kale (Tuscan cabbage) leaves

2 tbsp olive oil

2 tbsp balsamic vinegar

1 Preheat the oven to 230°C/450°F/gas 8.

2 Place the chopped squash, beetroot, and Brussels

Sprouts into a baking tray, drizzle over the coconut oil (if your kitchen is cool you may need to melt the coconut oil first by standing the jar in hot water) and toss to coat. Cook for 45 minutes, until the veggies are tender.

3 While the veggies are cooking, remove the kale leaves from the stem and tear into small bite-size pieces. Add to a large bowl.

4 Combine the olive oil and balsamic vinegar in a small bowl and set aside.

5 When the veggies are done cooking, add them to the kale and toss well, then add the dressing and toss again. Serve warm.

Watermelon Mint Salad

Summer

R ⏱

➕ Heart disease, diabetes, cancer, osteoporosis, migraines, vision, immunity, memory, GI, menstrual/PMS/menopause/PCOS

Serves 2

Nutrition per serving: 340kCal; 1421kJ; 7g protein; 54g carbohydrates; 15g fat; 2g saturated fat; 8g fibre; 36g sugar; 95mg salt

4 large handfuls of spinach leaves

¼ watermelon, cut into small cubes

1 large handful of fresh mint

4oz/110g/½ cup sugar snap peas, cut into bite-size pieces

2 tbsp olive oil

juice and zest of 1 lime

1 tbsp lime zest

1 Put the spinach, watermelon, mint and sugar snap peas into a large bowl.

2 In a separate bowl, combine the olive oil, lime juice and lime zest and mix well. Pour the

dressing over the salad ingredients and toss well to combine.

3 Serve chilled.

Soups

Creamy Parsnip Soup

Autumn/Winter

R

✚ Heart disease, cancer, allergies, immunity, liver, gall bladder

Serves 6

Nutrition per serving: 210kCal; 878kJ; 3g protein; 41g carbohydrates; 5g fat; 1g saturated fat; 9g fibre; 15g sugar; 170mg salt

1 head of garlic

2 tbsp olive oil, plus a drizzle

1 large white onion, diced

2 celery stalks, diced

½ tsp kosher salt

1¾lbs/900g parsnips, peeled and chopped into 2in/5cm chunks

1 large red (russet) potato, peeled and chopped into 2in/5cm chunks

4¼ pints/1.5 litres/6 cups low-sodium vegetable stock

3 bay leaves

kosher salt and freshly ground white pepper, to taste

paprika, for dusting

1 Preheat the oven to 200°C/400°F/gas 6.

2 Cut the top off the head of garlic, exposing the cloves. Place cut side up on a piece of aluminium foil. Drizzle the exposed cloves with a bit of olive oil, then wrap the foil over the garlic head and seal, making a package. Place in the oven and roast for 25 minutes.

3 Unwrap the foil and let the garlic cool. When cool enough to handle, squeeze the softened cloves out of their skins. Set aside 6 cloves for the soup and refrigerate the rest for another use.

4 While the garlic is cooking, heat the olive oil in a large pan over a medium heat. Add the onion, celery and salt and sauté until the vegetables are soft and translucent, about 5 minutes.

5 Add the parsnips, potato, vegetable stock and bay leaves and bring to a boil. Reduce the heat, cover and simmer until the vegetables are very soft, about 45 minutes.

6 Remove the bay leaves and let the soup cool slightly. Transfer the soup to a blender. Add the roasted garlic cloves and purée (be careful – the soup is hot!) or add the roasted garlic to the pot and purée with an immersion blender. Season with the kosher salt and white pepper to taste.

7 To serve, portion the soup into bowls and dust with the paprika.

Cauliflower Soup

Winter/Spring

R ⊙

✚ Heart disease, cancer, allergies, auto-immune conditions,
liver, gall bladder

Serves 4

Nutrition per serving: 120kCal; 502kJ; 3g protein; 13g
carbohydrates; 7g fat; 1g saturated fat; 4g fibre; 6g sugar; 480mg
salt

> 32fl oz/1 litre/4 cups low-sodium vegetable
> broth
>
> 1 head of cauliflower, cut into small florets
>
> 2 tbsp extra virgin olive oil
>
> 1 yellow onion, chopped
>
> coconut or olive oil, for sautéing
>
> dash of Himalayan salt and freshly ground
> black pepper, to taste

1 Bring the vegetable broth to a boil in a large
   pan, then add the cauliflower florets and the
   olive oil and cook for at least 10 minutes, until
   soft.

2 While the cauliflower is cooking, sauté the onion

in coconut or olive oil until translucent, about 5 minutes.

3 When cooked, transfer to a blender in batches and purée or use an immersion blender.

4 Return to the pan and heat the soup for a few minutes.

5 Serve in small bowls. Add a drizzle of olive oil (optional) and a sprinkle of Himalayan salt and pepper, to taste.

Summertime Watermelon Gazpacho

Summer

R

✛ Heart disease, stroke, cancer, arthritis, migraines, inflammation/pain, thyroid, weight loss, skin, PCOS/menstrual

Serves 6

Nutrition per serving: 168 kCal; 703 kJ; 3 g protein; 18 g carbohydrates; 11 g fat; 1 g saturated fat; 3 g fibre; 12 g sugar; 200 mg salt

Soup:

24oz/675g/4½ cups seedless watermelon, coarsely chopped

24oz/675g/4½ cups ripe summer tomatoes, diced

2 cucumbers, peeled and coarsely chopped

1 handful fresh basil leaves, coarsely chopped

4 tablespoons olive oil

¼ red onion, coarsely chopped

2 garlic cloves, coarsely chopped

2 tablespoons red wine vinegar

1½ teaspoons Himalayan salt

½ teaspoon whole cumin seeds (optional)

⅛ teaspoon cayenne pepper (optional)

Garnish:

1.5oz/40g/½ cup cucumber, diced

2.5oz/70g/½ cup diced
seedless watermelon

Fresh basil

Olive oil

1 Toss all ingredients in large bowl until evenly coated and allow to marinate for 20 minutes.

2 Add the mixture to a blender in batches and puree, or use an immersion blender, adding water to get your preferred consistency.

3 Place in refrigerator for at least 30 minutes before serving.

4 Serve chilled with suggested garnish.

Thank you to Reboot success story Angela Von Buelow, co-host of JuicingRadio.com, for this recipe.

Fierce Carrot Avocado Soup

Summer

R ⏲

✚ Heart disease, stroke, cancer, arthritis, migraines, inflammation/pain, thyroid, skin, immunity, vision

Serves 4

Nutrition per serving: 290Cal; 1214kJ; 6g protein; 52g carbohydrates; 8g fat; 1g saturated fat; 14g fibre; 17g sugar; 450mg salt

20fl oz/500ml/2½ cups fresh organic carrot juice

2 avocados, peeled

1 tablespoon fresh ginger, minced

1 garlic clove, chopped

¼ tsp cayenne (or more to taste)

1 tpsp lemon juice

1 jalapeño pepper, seeded

5 fresh sweet mint leaves

15-20 basil leaves

pinch of pink Himalayan salt

1 Reserving half an avocado, place all the ingredients in a blender and puree until smooth. Adjust seasoning to taste. This soup is delicious at room temperature or slightly chilled.

2 Garnish with sliced avocado and a mint or basil leaf.

Thank you to Reboot success story Angela Von Buelow, co-host of JuicingRadio.com, for this recipe.

Spicy Roots Soup

Autumn/Winter

R ⏱ 🏃

✚ Heart disease, cancer, arthritis, gout, allergies, migraines,
inflammation/pain, auto-immune conditions, weight loss/
obesity, vision, immunity, liver, menstrual/PMS/menopause/
PCOS, gall bladder

Serves 6

Nutrition per serving: 250kCal; 1045kJ; 6g protein; 29g
carbohydrates; 13g fat; 2g saturated fat; 7g fibre; 10g sugar;
190mg salt

2 tbsp olive oil

1 large sweet onion, diced

1 leek chopped

5 garlic cloves, peeled and chopped

1 large sweet potato, cubed

2 large parsnips, peeled and chopped

5 large carrots, peeled and chopped

¼ chilli pepper (jalapeño), diced (optional)

1 tbsp curry powder

1 tsp turmeric

4in/10cm piece of fresh root ginger, peeled
and grated

3 tbsp fresh sage, chopped

black pepper to taste

48fl oz/1.5 litre/6 cups low-sodium
   vegetable broth

1 Heat the olive oil in a heavy pot over a medium heat. Sauté the onion, leek and garlic until softened but not browned, about 5 minutes.

2 Add the sweet potato, parsnips, carrots, chilli pepper and spices, and then the vegetable broth and water. Cover and simmer until the vegetables are soft (your fork should be able to easily pierce through), about 30 minutes.

3 Transfer to a blender in batches and purée or use an immersion blender.

4 Add soup back into pot and warm on a medium heat for a few minutes.

5 Serve warm.

Sides

Pear and Roasted Brussels Sprouts

Autumn/Winter

R ☉ 🏃

✚ Heart disease, stroke, high cholesterol, cancer, osteoporosis, arthritis, inflammation/pain, weight loss/obesity, immunity, memory, GI, liver, menstrual/PMS/menopause/PCOS

Serves 2

Nutrition per serving: 180kCal; 334kJ; 6g protein; 29g carbohydrates; 3.5g fat; 0g saturated fat; 8g fibre; 14g sugar; 70mg salt

7oz/200g/2 cups Brussels sprouts, halved

½ medium pear, cut into small cubes

1 tsp olive oil

1 tbsp dried cranberries

dash of salt and freshly ground pepper, to taste

1 Preheat the oven to 220°C/425°F/gas 7.

2 Place the Brussels sprouts and pear in a glass baking dish lined with aluminium foil. Add the olive oil, salt and pepper.

3 Roast in the oven for about 25 minutes, stirring the mixture every 5–10 minutes, until the Brussels sprouts are tender and brown. Remove from the oven, add the cranberries, and serve!

Caprese Kale Sauté

Summary

R ⊙ ☀

✚ Heart disease, stroke, high cholesterol, diabetes, cancer, osteoporosis, gout, allergies, migraines, auto-immune conditions, vision, skin, immunity, memory, liver, menstrual/ PMS/menopause/PCOS, gall bladder

Serves 2

Nutrition per serving: 60kCal; 251kJ; 3g protein; 9g carbohydrates; 3g fat; 0g saturated fat; 2g fibre; 1g sugar; 30mg salt

3 tsps olive oil

2 garlic cloves, chopped

4oz/110g/½ cup cherry tomatoes, halved

14oz/450g/2 cups kale (Tuscan cabbage) leaves

½ tsp dried basil

dash of sea salt and pepper to taste

1 Warm a sauté pan over a medium heat and add the olive oil. Sautée the tomatoes for about 5 minutes and then add the garlic. Cook for a further 3 minutes, until fragrant.

2 Add the kale to the pan, stir and cover. Continue to cook for about 5 minutes or until the kale is cooked but not wilted. Add the basil, salt and pepper to the pan and mix well to combine.

3 Remove the pan from the heat and serve immediately.

Garam Masala Spring (Collard) Greens

Spring

R

✚ Cancer, arthritis, weight loss, inflammation/pain, diabetes, PCOS, vision, skin, immunity , liver, osteoporosis, GI

Serves 2

Nutrition per serving: 370Cal; 1003kJ; 11g protein; 26g carbohydrates; 4g fat; 0g saturated fat; 16g fibre; 2g sugar; 90mg salt

2 bunches spring (collard) greens, chopped and ribs removed

1½ tsp Garam Masala

1 tsp turmeric

4 tbsp olive oil or coconut oil

2 tbsp mustard seed oil

1 tsp. sea salt or Himalayan salt

6 tbsp fresh coriander (cilantro), chopped

1 Heat a large saucepan or oven over medium high heat and add the garam masala and turmeric and heat for about 2 minutes until fragrant, stirring to make sure that the spices do not burn.

Add the olive oil and mustard oil to the pan, stirring until mixed.

2 Add the collard greens and salt and toss to coat with the oil. Cover the pan and cook until the greens are wilted, about 5 minutes.

3 Remove from the heat, mix in the chopped cilantro, then serve.

*Garam masala: Store bought or as follows

    2 tbsp cumin seeds

    2 tbsp coriander seeds

    2 tbsp cardamom

    1 tsp whole cloves

    2 tbsp black peppercorns

    1 small cinnamon stick

Grind all ingredients in a spice grinder or using a mortar and pestle.

Garlic Cauliflower Mash

Winter/Spring

R ⊙ ⅄

✚ arthritis, allergies, migraines, inflammation/pain, auto-immune
conditions, weight loss/obesity, immunity, memory, liver, gall
bladder

Serves 4

Nutrition per serving: 100kCal; 418kJ; 2g protein; 9g
carbohydrates; 7g fat; 3g saturated fat; 3g fibre; 4g sugar; 50mg
salt

1 head of cauliflower, cut into small florets

1 tbsp olive oil

2 garlic cloves, chopped

2 tbsp coconut oil

1 tsp fresh chives, chopped

1 tsp paprika

½ tsp each of sea salt and freshly ground
black pepper

1 Preheat the oven to 220°C/425°F/gas 7.

2 Place the cauliflower on a baking sheet lined
with parchment paper. Drizzle with olive oil
and add a pinch of salt and pepper. Place in

the oven and roast for 20 minutes until slightly browned.

3 Purée the roasted cauliflower, garlic, coconut oil and the remaining salt and pepper in a blender or food processor.

4 Serve garnished with chives and a sprinkle of paprika.

Crispy Kale Chips

Winter/Spring/Summer/Autumn

R ⊙

✚ Heart disease, stroke, high cholesterol, diabetes, cancer, osteoporosis, gout, allergies, migraines, inflammation/ pain, vision, skin, immunity, memory, liver, menstrual/PMS/ menopause/PCOS, gall bladder

Serves 4

Nutrition per serving: 90kCal; 376kJ; 2g protein; 7g carbohydrates; 7g fat; 1g saturated fat; 1g fibre; 0g sugar; 200mg salt

1 bunch of kale (Tuscan cabbage) leaves, stems removed and torn into large pieces

2 tbsp olive oil

sea salt, to taste

1 Preheat the oven to 150°C/300°F/gas 2.

2 Toss the kale and olive oil together in a large bowl; sprinkle with salt.

3 Spread on a baking sheet in a single layer and bake for 15 minutes or until crisp.

Mains

Sweet Potato Sliders

Autumn/Winter

R

✚ Heart disease, stroke, cancer, arthritis, migraines, allergies, skin, immunity, vision

Serves 3

Nutrition per serving: 140kCal; 586kJ; 2g protein; 16g carbohydrates; 9g fat; 1.5g saturated fat; 4g fibre; 4g sugar; 30mg salt

2 sweet potatoes, peeled and cut into circles (you need at least 24 slices)

12 baby Portobello mushrooms

sea salt and black pepper, to taste

Optional herbs (fresh when possible or dried): basil, oregano, old bay, cinnamon, cumin, chipotle, cracked red pepper

2 tsp olive oil

Spread

1 avocado

1 tbsp olive oil

1 tbsp water

2 garlic cloves

¼ onion

¼ teaspoon fresh ground black pepper

pinch sea salt (optional)

squeeze of lime

To serve

¼ cucumber, sliced

1 tomato, sliced

¼ red onion, sliced

2 kale leaves, chopped

1 Preheat oven to 220°C/425°F/gas 7.

2 Place the sweet potato slices onto a baking sheet and drizzle with 1 teaspoon of olive oil and half of the herbs. Bake for about 30–35 minutes, flipping about halfway through, until the sweet potato is cooked through but still slightly firm. Leave to cool.

3 Meanwhile, remove the stems from the mushrooms and place mushroom caps on a second baking tray. Drizzle with the remaining oil and herbs and bake for 10–15 minutes, until tender. Allow the mushrooms cool and drain on a paper towel, stem side down.

4 While the vegetables are cooking, place the spread ingredients in a blender or food processor until well combined.

5 Spoon spread onto 1 sweet potato circle. Add mushroom and top with other veggies – kale/lettuce, cucumber, tomato, onion, like a burger. Add a little more avocado spread and finally top with another sweet potato circle. Repeat the process until you've used all your sweet potatoes. You will most likely end up with leftover spread which goes well with carrots, celery and peppers.

Courgette (Zucchini) Noodles with Fresh & Easy Herb Tomato Sauce

Summary

Summer

R ⊙ 🏃

✚ Heart disease, high cholesterol, cancer, gout, inflammation/
pain, auto-immune conditions, weight loss/obesity, vision,
skin, memory, GI, liver, gall bladder

Serves 4

Nutrition per serving: 210kCal; 878kJ; 6g protein; 20g carbohydrates; 15g fat; 2g saturated fat; 6g fibre; 12g sugar; 45mg salt

4 courgettes (zucchini)

2 tbsp olive oil

Sauce:

2 tbsp olive oil

1 onion, chopped

10 tomatoes, chopped

4 garlic cloves, chopped

1 handful fresh parsley, chopped

1 tsp ground cumin

1 tbsp dried oregano

1 tbsp dried thyme

sea salt (about ½ tsp) and freshly ground
pepper (½–1 tsp), to taste

Tip: a spiralizer is a tool that is used to make long ribbons from
vegetables – you can pick one up at a cooking store. If you don't own
a spiralizer, you can slice the courgette in a food processor, or with a
mandolin, or use a sharp knife to make thin strips.

1 Slice the courgettes in half and assemble one half
at a time on the spiralizer. Push them through
and allow the noodles to fall into a bowl. Cut the
noodles into sizes that you prefer.

2 Heat the olive oil in a large pan over a medium-
low heat. Add courgette noodles and cook until
soft, about 5–10 minutes. You don't have to heat
them but it will soften them. Drain the noodles
before adding your tomato sauce.

3 Meanwhile, heat 2 tbsp olive oil in an iron skillet
or an oven-safe pan on a low-medium heat. Add
the onion and sauté until soft, 11–13 minutes. Add
the tomatoes, garlic, spices, herbs, salt and pepper
to the onions. Simmer on low-medium heat for
5–8 minutes.

4 Serve the tomato sauce over the courgette
noodles.

Tomato-Basil Spaghetti Squash

Autumn

R

✚ Heart disease, stroke, high cholesterol, cancer, osteoporosis,
arthritis, gout, auto-immune conditions, skin, immunity,
memory, GI, menstrual/PMS/menopause/PCOS

Serves 2

Nutrition per serving: 180kCal; 752kJ; 6g protein; 31g
carbohydrates; 6g fat; 1g saturated fat; 8g fibre; 15g sugar; 690mg
salt

1 medium or large spaghetti squash, cut in
   half and seeds removed

1 tsp olive oil

½ medium yellow onion, chopped

1 garlic clove, chopped

1–2 medium broccoli heads, chopped

5oz/150g/¾ cup cherry tomatoes, halved

4fl oz/120ml/½ cup organic tomato sauce
   (passata)

sea salt and freshly ground pepper, to taste

fresh basil leaves, to garnish

1 Preheat the oven to 180°C/350°F/gas 4.

2 Place the squash halves face down onto a baking sheet lightly coated with olive oil. Cook in the oven for about 1 hour or until soft. Remove the squash from the oven and allow to cool.

3 Heat the olive oil in a medium pan. Add the onion and garlic and cook for about 5 minutes or until soft. Add the broccoli and cherry tomatoes and continue to cook, stirring occasionally until the vegetables are soft. Add the tomato sauce and simmer for 5 minutes, stirring occasionally.

4 Scoop the insides of the spaghetti squash into the hot pan using a fork. Fold the squash into the ingredients in the pan to coat with sauce, and add the salt and pepper. Serve garnished with fresh basil.

Baked Courgette (Zucchini) with Herbs

Summer

R

+ High-cholesterol, cancer, gout, inflammation/pain, auto-immune conditions, thyroid, weight loss/obesity, vision, skin, immunity, GI, menstrual/PMS/menopause/PCOS

Serves 4

Nutrition per serving: 190 kCal; 795 kJ; 4 g protein; 13 g carbohydrates; 14 g fat; 2 g saturated fat; 4 g fibre; 9 g sugar; 45 mg salt

5 courgettes (zucchini)

4 spring onions (scallions), chopped, white and green parts separated

1 onion, chopped

2 plum tomatoes, chopped and deseeded

2 tbsp celery leaves (from inner stalks), chopped

4 tbsp basil leaves, chopped, plus extra for garnish

4oz/125ml/¼ cup olive oil

1 tsp sea salt

½ tsp fresh ground black pepper

1 Preheat oven to 220 / 425 / gas mark 7.

2 Slice the courgettes in half crosswise. Cut each half lengthwise, and cut or mandolin into ¼in/5mm sticks.

3 In a bowl, mix together the courgettes with the white parts of the spring onions, onion, tomatoes, celery leaves and basil. Mix in the olive oil, salt and pepper and toss to combine.

4 Pour into a baking dish and bake for 20 minutes.

5 Garnish with the remaining spring onions and chopped basil.

Stuffed Winter Pumpkin

✚ Heart disease, stroke, high cholesterol, cancer, osteoporosis, arthritis, allergies, inflammation/pain, vision, skin, immunity, memory, GI, liver, menstrual/PMS/Menopause/PCOS, gall bladder

Serves 2

Nutrition per serving: 200kCal; 836kJ; 8g protein; 33g carbohydrates; 6g fat; 1g saturated fat; 7g fibre; 11g sugar; 60mg salt

1 small to medium sugar pumpkin, top cut off and seeds removed

½ medium yellow onion, chopped

4oz/110g/½ cup cherry tomatoes, halved

1½oz/40g/½ cup sliced white or baby bella mushrooms

1 handful of spinach leaves

4 large Brussels sprouts, halved

½ tsp dried basil

olive oil, to drizzle

sea salt and freshly ground black pepper, to taste

1 Preheat the oven to 350°F/180°C/gas 4.

2 Place the onions, tomatoes, mushrooms, spinach and Brussels sprouts in a mixing bowl. Drizzle with olive oil, sprinkle with salt and pepper and scatter over the basil. Stuff all the ingredients into the pumpkin.

3 Place the stuffed pumpkin on a baking sheet lined with baking parchment and transfer to the oven. Check the pumpkin after 90 minutes to see if the vegetables are bubbling and the flesh of the pumpkin is soft. The pumpkin should be completely cooked in approximately 2 hours. Serve warm.

Pulp

A note of caution: not all these recipes are Reboot-friendly. If you are on a Reboot, try freezing your pulp and making these when you've finished your Reboot.

Homemade Pulp Vegetable Broth

R

+ cancer, arthritis, inflammation/pain, weight loss/obesity, immunity, GI

Serves 6

Nutrition per serving: 20 kCal; 84 kJ; 3 g protein; 10 g carbohydrates; 2 g fat; 0 g saturated fat; 5 g fibre; 2 g sugar; 15 mg salt

1 tsp olive oil

Pulp from making 2 of the juice recipes in this book

96fl oz/2½ litres/12 cups water

fresh or dried herbs: chives, thyme,
   rosemary, oregano, basil, bay leaves, use
   any herbs you like (try including ginger,
   parsley, etc.)

½ tsp each sea salt and freshly ground
   black pepper

1 Heat the olive oil in a pan over a medium heat.
  Add the pulp and stir for 1–2 minutes. Add the
  water, herbs, spices and seasonings and turn up
  to a high heat. Bring to a boil, then reduce the
  heat and simmer, uncovered, for 2–3 hours.

2 Strain with a fine mesh colander or sieve over
  a bowl.

3 Leave to cool, then sip and enjoy!

Note: Use in soup recipes. Also Vegetable Broth
is a great substitute to water or tea when Rebooting.
And it's great on a cold day!

Thai Infused Vegetable Broth

🕐 🏃

✚ Exercise, pain/inflammation, immunity, weight loss, diabetes, PCOS, arthritis, thyroid, immunity

Serves 6

Nutrition per serving: 28 kCal; 105 kJ; 1 g protein; 7 g carbohydrates; 1 g fat; 0 g saturated fat; 0 g fibre; 0 g sugar; 3 mg salt

10oz/300g/2 cups of vegetable pulp (weight of pulp will vary depending on the efficiency of your juicer)

64 fl oz/2 litres/8 cups of water

2 sticks of lemongrass, chopped finely

2 garlic clove, crushed

fresh coriander (cilantro), chopped

sea salt and pepper, to taste

1–2 fresh chillies, chopped (optional)

1 Bring the water to the boil in a large pot, then turn down the heat and add the pulp, lemongrass, garlic, coriander, chilli, salt and pepper.

2 Simmer, covered, for 2 hours.

3 Strain through a fine mesh colander or sieve over a bowl.

4 Leave to cool, then sip and enjoy! Vegetable broth is a great substitute for water or tea when Rebooting. And great on a cold day.

Black Bean Quinoa Veggie Pulp Burgers

✚ Heart disease, stroke, high cholesterol, diabetes,
osteoporosis, arthritis, gout, allergies, inflammation/pain,
weight loss/obesity, skin, GI, liver, gall bladder

Serves 6

Nutrition per serving: 232 kCal; 971 kJ; 9 g protein; 12 g
carbohydrates; 5 g fat; 1 g saturated fat; 7 g fibre; 16 g sugar;
59 mg salt

4½oz/125g/½ cup quinoa

8fl oz/225ml/1 cup water (for the quinoa)

1 can (6oz/450g) BPA-free black beans

4oz/100g/1 cup pulp (weight of pulp will
    depend on the efficiency of your juicer)
    – use any variety, but carrot and kale is a
    great place to start

3oz/80g/½ cup rolled oats

1 tsp dried chilli pepper

1 tsp ground cumin

½ tsp cayenne pepper

small handful of fresh coriander (cilantro)

1 tbsp olive oil

1 tsp coconut oil, for coating

1 avocado, sliced

juice of 1 lime

sea salt and freshly ground pepper, to taste

1 Preheat the oven to 230°C/450°F/gas 8.

2 Put the quinoa and water in a pan and bring to a boil. Reduce to a simmer and stir occasionally. Cook for about 15 minutes, until all the water is evaporated.

3 While the quinoa is cooking, rinse and drain the black beans well. Combine the beans, cooked quinoa, juice pulp, oats, chilli pepper, cumin, cayenne, coriander, salt, pepper and olive oil in a large bowl and mix well. You can lightly mash the mixture as you stir it to make it stick together. Once well combined, make the mixture into 6 small patties.

4 Coat a baking sheet with a light layer of coconut oil, place the patties on the pan, drizzle them with a little oil and bake for 12 minutes. The burgers might be a bit crispy on the outside, so cook them shorter or longer depending on your preference.

5 Once cooked, top with slices of avocado and a squeeze of fresh lime juice.

Veggie Meatballs

🕐 🏃

➕ Heart disease, diabetes, cancer, arthritis, gout, allergies, inflammation/pain, auto-immune conditions, thyroid, skin, memory, liver, gall bladder

Serves 2

Nutrition per serving: 298 kCal; 1247 kJ; 6 g protein; 19 g carbohydrates; 14 g fat; 1 g saturated fat; 7 g fibre; 15 g sugar; 20 mg salt

4oz/100g/1 cup pulp (weight of pulp will vary depending on the efficiency of your juicer) from kale, spinach, celery, cucumber, carrots, apple

½ sweet red (bell) pepper (capsicum), chopped

1 courgette (zucchini), chopped

2 garlic cloves, chopped

1 tbsp olive oil

1 tbsp fresh parsley, chopped

¾ tbsp Italian seasoning or dried oregano

3 tbsp ground flaxseed mixed with 8 tbsp water (for binding)

1oz/30g/¼ cup Nutritional Yeast (optional)

1 Preheat the oven to 180°C/350°F/gas 4.

2 Sauté the chopped vegetables in the olive oil over a medium heat. Transfer to a bowl. Mix the parsley, seasoning and pulp with the sautéed vegetables and add the flaxseed/water mixture plus Italian seasoning or oregano.

3 Form the mixture into balls, then place them on a baking dish. Sprinkle with Nutritional Yeast, if using, and place the dish in the oven. Cook until golden brown, about 15 minutes.

4 Add to your favourite whole wheat, wholegrain or spinach spaghetti and combine with a marinara sauce.

Banana, Carrot and Courgette (Zucchini) Muffins

R ⏱ 🏃

✚ Heart disease, stroke, high cholesterol, diabetes, arthritis, gout, allergies, inflammation/pain, auto-immune conditions, thyroid, vision, skin, immunity, memory

Makes 4–6 large muffins or 8–10 small ones

Nutrition per serving: 223 kCal; 933 kJ; 4 g protein; 19 g carbohydrates; 4 g fat; 1 g saturated fat; 6 g fibre; 15 g sugar; 65 mg salt

3 flax eggs (3 tbsp ground flaxseeds added to 9 tbsp of water and stirred),* or use 3 regular eggs

1oz/30g/¼ cup coconut flour

2 fresh bananas

4oz/100g/1 cup pulp (weight of pulp will vary depending on the efficiency of your juicer) from juiced carrots and courgette (zucchini)

¼ cup coconut oil

4 dates, pitted

½ tsp bicarbonate of soda (baking soda)

½ tsp sea salt

2oz/60g/½ cup walnuts, chopped

1 Preheat the oven to 180°C/350°F/gas 4.

2 Combine the flax eggs (or regular eggs), bananas, pulp, coconut oil and dates in a high-powered blender and blend until smooth. Add in the coconut flour, bicarbonate of soda, and salt and blend until smooth. Then fold in the walnuts.

3 Pour the mixture into a muffin pan (either grease the pan or spoon the mixture into muffin cases). Bake in the oven for 30–35 minutes.

4 Remove from oven and let sit for at least 20 minutes before serving. Slice in half and serve with your favourite nut butter, mashed-up berries or just alone!

* **NOTE**: These are easy to make gluten free muffins and will not rise as much as gluten muffins. The flax eggs will make the muffins even more cake-like and moist.

Rosemary Carrot Flax Crackers

🕐 🏃

➕ Heart disease, high cholesterol, diabetes, arthritis, migraines, inflammation/pain, auto-immune conditions, thyroid, vision, skin, immunity, memory, liver, menstrual/PMS/menopause/PCOS, gall bladder

Makes about 60 small crackers (serving size 10 crackers)

Nutrition per serving: 300 kCal; 1255 kJ; 8 g protein; 29 g carbohydrates; 22 g fat; 1 g saturated fat; 8 g fibre; 20 g sugar; 43 mg salt

4oz/110g/1 cup raw flax seeds

16oz/250g/4 cups raw sunflower seeds

4oz/100g/1 cup carrot pulp (weight of pulp will vary depending on the efficiency of your juicer)

1oz/30g/¼ cup raw sesame seeds

1 tbsp garlic powder

2 tbsp dried rosemary

1 tsp sea salt and freshly ground pepper, to taste

1 avocado (optional, to use as a spread on the crackers)

1 Combine the flax seeds with 8fl oz/250ml/1 cup of water and let sit for 1 hour, until it forms a gooey consistency.

2 Place the sunflower seeds and carrot pulp in a food processor and pulse until well chopped.

3 Transfer the sunflower seeds and pulp into a bowl and add the gooey flax seeds, then stir in the sesame seeds, garlic powder, rosemary, salt and pepper. Mix well until combined in a wet, crumbly mixture.

4 Spread in a thin layer on dehydrator trays lined with parchment paper. Score the crackers before dehydrating them so they snap apart easily and evenly when they are done. Leave to dehydrate for 7–8 hours at 115°F/46°C. *

5 Serve plain or add avocado as a healthy spread.

* **NOTE:** Don't have a dehydrator? Use your oven! Set your oven at its very lowest heat and leave your oven door open a crack. Place your crackers on a baking sheet lined with parchment paper and place in the oven. Leave the crackers to dry for at least 3–4 hours. Flip the crackers over and dry for another 30 minutes to 1 hour.

Healthy Dog Treats

15oz/450g/3 cups pulp (weight of pulp will vary depending on the efficiency of your juicer) from carrot, sweet potato, apple and spinach

5oz/125g/½ cup peanut butter

2oz/40g/¼ cup rolled oats

1 tbsp coconut oil

1 mashed banana

1 Preheat the oven to 180°C/350°F/gas 4.

2 Mix all the ingredients together until well combined, then roll into little cookie shapes – the size can vary depending on the size of your pet. Bake for 15 minutes.

3 Let cool before serving to your pet!

Resources

Need inspiration for how to eat post-Reboot? There are plenty of great plant-based, raw, vegetarian, Vegan, paleo and plant-based books available, check out the cooking section in any bookstore for ideas. If you want some recommendations, though, the following books are from authors who have been particularly inspiring to Rebooters. And don't forget, the Reboot Team is continually publishing new recipes on www.rebootwithjoe.com, so make sure to visit us!

- **Eat to Live Cookbook by Dr Joel Fuhrman** – filled with excellent plant-powered recipes to maintain your good health after a Reboot.

- **Eating on the Wild Side by Jo Robinson** – a great resource for getting the most nutrition and flavour out of your produce, full of tips on best varieties, storage and preparation.

- **Everyday Raw by Matthew Kenney** – any book from

chef Matthew Kenney is sure to be great. This one in particular is a great guide to raw 'cooking'.

- **Giada's Feel Good Food by Giada De Laurentiis** – full of practical, delicious recipes for all diet types including gluten-free, vegan, vegetarian and pescetarian.

- **It's All Good by Gwyneth Paltrow** – great recipes, mainly vegan, plus some pescetarian.

- **Living Raw Food by Sarma Melngailis** – food so good you won't believe it's all raw! From one of my favourite NYC restaurants, Pure.

- **Main Street Vegan by Victoria Moran** – complete guide to making the dietary and lifestyle shift to a vegan diet with simple, practical steps.

For your doctor

You might like to download a PDF of the following text to give to your doctor (visit www.rebootwithjoe.com/for-your-doctor):

Most medical experts agree on, and numerous studies show, the benefits of consuming fresh fruits and vegetables and fresh expressed juices in the prevention and treatment of obesity, cardiovascular disease, inflammatory conditions and cancer.

Your patient has expressed interest in starting the pathway towards healthier eating by participating in a Reboot programme. It is recommended that anyone with medical problems, on prescription medications, or who is interested in participating in the programme for longer than 15 days should consult with their doctor.

What is a Reboot?

- It is a chance to break the cycle of unhealthy eating.

- It is a temporary period of time in which a person commits to eating and/or drinking only fruits and vegetables.

- It is not a diet; it is a time for the body and mind to reset and maximally absorb micronutrients and phytonutrients to allow for a transition to healthier wholefoods and plant-rich eating behaviours.

Why include juice?

How many patients have told you they would eat more vegetables, but they just don't like the taste? Juicing overcomes this obstacle. It offers many delicious health benefits, including numerous servings of fruits and veggies in just one glass, full of immune-boosting nutrients and phytochemicals naturally found in freshly extracted juice. Most commercial juices are highly processed and lack nutrition compared to freshly juiced fruits and vegetables.

Reboot basics

- Reboot length can vary from 3 to 60 days.

- Guidelines are provided online to help individuals decide which Reboot programme is best for them, and all the information needed is available free of charge at www.rebootwithjoe.com.

- Individual and group support from credentialed nutritionists from respected academic institutions is available in Guided Reboots for a reasonable fee.

- Fruits and vegetables are the principal components of a Reboot, followed by guidelines for other healthy food choices after the completion of a Reboot.

- Many people find that replacing breakfast and lunch with a nutrient-packed fresh fruit juice or smoothie, along with a healthy dinner, results in significant improvements in eating habits, health and weight.

Protein

A Reboot is not meant to be a long-term meal plan. Plant-based protein is present in the foods eaten during a Reboot. Because this is a short-term change designed ultimately to lead to healthier eating habits, protein deficiencies do not typically develop. If you have concerns about your patient's protein intake during a Reboot, we have several plant-based protein supplements that we can recommend adding into their plan.

Medical support

- Medical judgement with regard to each individual patient is left to the discretion of the treating doctor.

- In general, no laboratory studies are recommended for healthy individuals completing a programme of up to 15 days.

- Although we have not seen any participants develop electrolyte abnormalities, we recommend that doctors check electrolytes every 15 days in those healthy individuals who are doing a juice-only Reboot for longer than 15 days.

- A juice-only Reboot is not recommended for more than 60 days, and the length of time is in part based on the BMI of the individual.

- Healthy individuals on anti-hypertensive medications have also participated in Reboots for extended periods of time, and we recommend electrolytes be checked in these individuals every 10 days. Many individuals on anti-hypertensives have been able to decrease their doses or discontinue the usage of some medications as their blood pressure normalises. It is recommended to monitor a patient's blood pressure during and after a Reboot and adjust their medications as needed.

- Patients with diabetes have also successfully participated in both juice-only and juice-plus-food Reboots, leading to decreasing and sometimes eliminating the need for medications. It is not recommended that anyone with diabetes participate without a doctor's or nutritionist's guidance.

If you have additional questions about the use of a Reboot for your patients, please email info@rebootwithjoe.com and our nutritionists or physicians from the Medical Advisory Board will contact you. Please note that this service is intended for doctors only; due to the volume of emails we do not respond to questions from individuals.

Free online support is provided to anyone interested in participating in a Reboot at www.rebootwithjoe.com.

Notes

1 "Preventable illness makes up approximately 70 per cent of the burden of illness and the associated costs. Well-developed national statistics such as those outlined in Healthy People 2000, Health U.S. 1991, and elsewhere document this central fact clearly."

    James F. Fries, C. Everett Koop, Carson E. Beadle, Paul P. Cooper, Mary Jane England, Roger F. Greaves, Jacque J. Sokolov, Daniel Wright, and the Health Project Consortium, "Reducing Health Care Costs by Reducing the Need and Demand for Medical Services." *New England Journal of Medicine* 329 (July 29, 1993): 321–325.

2 John P. Reganold et al., Bisphenol A and Risk of Metabolic Disorders, *The Journal of the American Medical Association*, 2008; 300(11): 1353–1355.

    Iain A. Lang, Tamara S. Galloway, Alan Scarlett et al., Association of Urinary Bisphenol A Concentration With Medical Disorders and Laboratory Abnormalities in Adults, *The Journal of the American Medical Association*, 2008; 300(11): 1303–1310.

'Our conclusions are consistent with the large number of hazards and adverse effects identified in laboratory animals exposed to low doses of BPA.' L. N. Vandenberg et al., Human exposures to bisphenol A: mismatches between data and assumptions, *Reviews on Environmental Health*, 2013; 28(1): 37–58.

3 http://organic-center.org/reportfiles/YieldsReport. pdf

4 http://www.plosone.org/article/ info%3Adoi%2F10.1371%2Fjournal. pone.0056354#pone.0056354-Foyer1

5 *'Eating on the Wild Side: The Missing Link to Optimum Health,* Jo Robinson, Little, Brown, 2013.

6 https://www.diabetes.org.uk/About_us/What- we-say/Statistics/Diabetes-prevalence-2012/

7 http://www.aihw.gov.au/diabetes/

Index

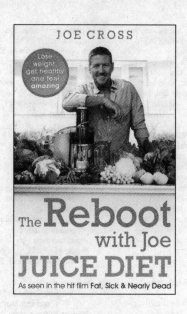

JOE CROSS

Lose weight, get healthy and feel amazing

The **Reboot** with Joe **JUICE DIET**

As seen in the hit film *Fat, Sick & Nearly Dead*

'When I made my film *Fat, Sick & Nearly Dead*, I literally <u>was</u> fat, sick and nearly dead. I was overweight, loaded up on steroids and suffering from an autoimmune disease. I knew I had to drastically change my lifestyle. So I traded in my junk food diet and only drank fresh fruit and vegetable juices for the next 60 days. I lost the weight, got myself off all medication and truly Rebooted my life. Now I could never imagine returning to my old ways again. And you know what? If I can do it, so can you!'

JOE CROSS

Joe has distilled all he's learned during his incredible journey of transformation into *The Reboot with Joe Juice Diet*. Now you too can take control of your diet and improve your health by consuming more fruits and vegetables. It really is that simple.

Available in trade paperback and ebook
www.hodder.co.uk